AF487907

The Human Body Unveiled

A Deep Dive into Anatomy and Physiology

Nancy Graves

© **Copyright 2024 by Nancy Graves**
All Rights Reserved

This document is geared towards providing exact and reliable information with regards to the topic and issue covered. The publication is sold with the idea that the publisher is not required to render accounting, officially permitted, or otherwise, qualified services. If advice is necessary, legal or professional, a practiced individual in the profession should be ordered. From a Declaration of Principles which was accepted and approved equally by a Committee of the American Bar Association and a Committee of Publishers and Associations. In no way is it legal to reproduce, duplicate, or transmit any part of this document in either electronic means or in printed format. Recording of this publication is strictly prohibited and any storage of this document is not allowed unless with written permission from the publisher. All rights reserved. The information provided herein is stated to be truthful and consistent, in that any liability, in terms of inattention or otherwise, by any usage or abuse of any policies, processes, or directions contained within is the solitary and after responsibility of the recipient reader. Under no circumstances will any legal responsibility or blame be held against the publisher for any reparation, damages, or monetary loss due to the information herein, either directly or indirectly. Respective authors own all copyrights not held by the publisher. The information herein is offered for informational purposes solely, and is universal as so.

The presentation of the information is without contract or any type of guarantee assurance. The trademarks that are used are without any consent, and the publication of the trademark is without permission or backing by the trademark owner. All trademarks and brands within this book are for clarifying purposes only and are the owned by the owners themselves, not affiliated with this document.

Table of Contents

Chapter 1

Introduction to Anatomy and Physiology

The Importance of Studying Anatomy and Physiology

Understanding the human body is a fundamental aspect of comprehending life itself. Anatomy and physiology are the twin pillars upon which this understanding is built, providing a detailed map and functional blueprint of the human body. This knowledge is not just the domain of healthcare professionals; it is essential for anyone interested in health, fitness, and the biological sciences. The importance of studying anatomy and physiology extends far beyond the classroom, impacting daily life, personal health, and even societal well-being.

One of the primary reasons for studying anatomy and physiology is to gain a clear and comprehensive understanding of how the body works. Anatomy, the study of the structure of body parts and their relationships to one another, provides a static map of the human body. Physiology, on the other hand, explores the dynamic processes and functions of these parts, explaining how they work individually and as systems. Together, they form a holistic view of the body, akin to understanding both the hardware and software of a complex machine. This foundational knowledge is crucial for identifying how different parts of the body interact and support each other.

An in-depth understanding of anatomy and physiology is indispensable for healthcare professionals. Doctors, nurses, therapists, and other medical practitioners rely on this knowledge to diagnose and treat illnesses. By comprehending the normal anatomy and physiology of the body, they can recognize when something is amiss and determine the most effective treatment. For example, understanding the intricacies of the cardiovascular system enables cardiologists to diagnose heart diseases and prescribe appropriate interventions. Similarly, knowledge of the musculoskeletal system helps orthopedic surgeons perform precise surgeries to repair injuries.

Beyond the medical field, knowledge of anatomy and physiology is beneficial for anyone interested in fitness and wellness. Personal trainers, coaches, and fitness enthusiasts use this understanding to optimize physical performance and prevent injuries. Knowing how muscles, bones, and joints function allows for the design of effective exercise programs that enhance strength, flexibility, and endurance. For instance, understanding the role of the core muscles can guide the development of exercises that improve stability and prevent lower back pain. Additionally, awareness of the body's metabolic processes can inform nutritional choices that support overall health and fitness goals.

Anatomy and physiology also play a crucial role in understanding and managing personal health. Individuals equipped with this knowledge can make informed decisions about their health and well-being. Recognizing the symptoms of common ailments and understanding the importance of preventive measures can lead to earlier interventions and better health outcomes. For example, knowing the signs of a stroke or heart attack can prompt immediate action, potentially saving lives. Similarly, understanding the body's response to stress can guide the adoption of relaxation techniques to maintain mental and physical health.

Moreover, studying anatomy and physiology fosters a deeper appreciation of the human body. The intricate design and remarkable functions of the body inspire awe and respect. This appreciation can lead to a more mindful and respectful approach to one's own body and health. For instance, understanding the body's need for rest and recovery can encourage better sleep habits and stress management practices. This holistic appreciation also extends to recognizing the interconnectedness of body systems and the impact of lifestyle choices on overall health.

In addition to personal benefits, the study of anatomy and physiology has broader societal implications. Public health initiatives often rely on this knowledge to develop effective strategies for disease prevention and health promotion. For example, understanding the transmission and effects of infectious diseases informs vaccination programs and hygiene practices. Similarly, knowledge of nutritional science and metabolic processes underpins dietary guidelines and public health campaigns aimed at reducing obesity and related diseases.

Education in anatomy and physiology also has the potential to drive scientific and medical advancements. Researchers and scientists use this foundational knowledge to explore new treatments, technologies, and therapies. Breakthroughs in medical science, such as the development of organ transplantation, gene therapy, and advanced surgical techniques, are rooted in a deep understanding of human anatomy and physiology. These advancements not only improve individual health outcomes but also enhance the quality of life for society as a whole.

Furthermore, the importance of studying anatomy and physiology extends to the ethical and empathetic dimensions of healthcare. A thorough understanding of the human body cultivates a sense of empathy and compassion in healthcare providers. Recognizing the physical and emotional experiences of patients fosters better patient care and communication. This empathetic approach is essential for building trust and rapport, ultimately leading to more effective and patient-centered care.

The study of anatomy and physiology also encourages critical thinking and problem-solving skills. The complexity of the human body and its functions requires a systematic and analytical approach to learning. Students and professionals must integrate knowledge from various disciplines, such as biology, chemistry, and physics, to understand how the body operates. This interdisciplinary approach enhances cognitive skills and prepares individuals for the complex and dynamic nature of healthcare and scientific research.

In the realm of education, teaching anatomy and physiology equips students with valuable skills and knowledge that extend beyond the sciences. The structured and detailed study of the human body promotes discipline, attention to detail, and perseverance. These qualities are transferable to other fields and endeavors, making students more well-rounded and capable individuals.

Historical Perspectives on Human Anatomy

The study of human anatomy, the science of understanding the structure of the human body, has roots that run deep through the annals of history. Tracing the historical perspectives on human anatomy reveals a fascinating journey of discovery, marked by curiosity, innovation, and sometimes controversy. From ancient civilizations to modern times, each era has contributed uniquely to our current understanding of the human body.

In ancient Egypt, one of the earliest recorded instances of anatomical study emerged. The Egyptians' meticulous practices in mummification around 3000 BCE provided them with a rudimentary understanding of the human body's internal structures. Their religious and spiritual beliefs necessitated the preservation of bodies for the afterlife, leading to detailed observations of organs such as the heart, liver, and lungs. The Edwin Smith Papyrus, an ancient Egyptian medical text dating back to around 1600 BCE, offers insights into their anatomical knowledge and surgical practices. Although their understanding was limited and intertwined with mythological interpretations, it laid the groundwork for future anatomical exploration.

The ancient Greeks significantly advanced anatomical knowledge through a more systematic and empirical approach. Hippocrates, often regarded as the father of medicine, emphasized the importance of direct observation and study of the human body. His teachings, compiled in the Hippocratic Corpus, advocated for a rational and natural explanation of diseases, moving away from supernatural beliefs. However, it was Herophilus and Erasistratus, Greek physicians of the Hellenistic period, who made groundbreaking contributions. Herophilus, often called the father of anatomy, conducted dissections on human cadavers in Alexandria around 300 BCE. He distinguished between veins and arteries, described the nervous system, and identified various organs and their functions. Erasistratus, his contemporary, furthered this work by studying the brain and the circulatory system. Despite the ethical and moral controversies surrounding dissection, their work laid a critical foundation for anatomical science.

During the Roman era, Galen of Pergamon emerged as a towering figure in anatomy and medicine. Living from 129 to around 200 CE, Galen was a prolific writer and physician whose works dominated medical knowledge for over a millennium. Although his dissections were primarily on animals due to societal restrictions on human dissection, Galen's extensive writings on anatomy, physiology, and pathology were highly influential. He described the functions of various organs, the circulatory system, and the importance of the brain. However, Galen's reliance on animal dissection led to several inaccuracies in his understanding of human anatomy. His authoritative texts, despite their errors, became the bedrock of medical education in medieval Europe and the Islamic world.

The Islamic Golden Age, spanning from the 8th to the 14th centuries, witnessed significant advancements in anatomical knowledge. Islamic scholars translated and preserved Greek and Roman medical texts, ensuring their survival through turbulent times. Avicenna, or Ibn Sina, was a Persian polymath whose monumental work, "The Canon of Medicine," synthesized and expanded upon classical medical knowledge. Avicenna's contributions to anatomy, although primarily based on Galenic texts, included detailed descriptions of the skeletal, muscular, and nervous systems. His work influenced both Islamic and European medicine for centuries.

The Renaissance period marked a revolutionary era in anatomical study, characterized by a return to direct observation and dissection. Andreas Vesalius, a Flemish anatomist, is often heralded as the father of modern anatomy. His seminal work, "De Humani Corporis Fabrica" (On the Fabric of the Human Body), published in 1543, challenged the prevailing Galenic doctrines. Vesalius conducted meticulous dissections on human cadavers, providing accurate and detailed illustrations of the human body. His insistence on empirical observation and direct study overturned many of Galen's inaccuracies and established anatomy as a rigorous scientific discipline.

The Renaissance also saw the contributions of other notable anatomists. Leonardo da Vinci, renowned for his artistic genius, was also an avid student of anatomy. His detailed anatomical drawings, based on dissections he performed, revealed an extraordinary understanding of the human body's structure. Although his anatomical work remained largely unpublished during his lifetime, it profoundly influenced subsequent anatomical studies.

The 17th and 18th centuries ushered in further advancements with the development of new techniques and tools. William Harvey's discovery of the circulatory system in the early 17th century revolutionized the understanding of blood flow and the heart's function. Harvey's meticulous experiments and observations demonstrated that blood circulates continuously through the body, challenging the long-held belief in Galenic physiology. The invention of the microscope by Antonie van Leeuwenhoek and Robert Hooke in the late 17th century opened new vistas in anatomical study, allowing scientists to explore the microscopic structures of tissues and cells.

The 19th and 20th centuries saw the establishment of anatomy as a formal scientific discipline, with significant contributions from various anatomists and medical professionals. Henry Gray's "Gray's Anatomy," first published in 1858, became a landmark reference work, providing comprehensive and accessible information on human anatomy. The book's detailed illustrations and clear descriptions made it an indispensable resource for medical students and practitioners.

The development of advanced imaging techniques in the 20th century, such as X-rays, computed tomography (CT), and magnetic resonance imaging (MRI), revolutionized the field of anatomy. These technologies allowed for non-invasive visualization of internal structures, enhancing diagnostic capabilities and expanding anatomical knowledge. The Human Genome Project, completed in 2003, further enriched the understanding of human anatomy by mapping the genetic blueprint of the human body.

In contemporary times, the study of anatomy continues to evolve, integrating new technologies and interdisciplinary approaches. Virtual dissection tools, three-dimensional imaging, and computer simulations have transformed anatomical education, providing interactive and immersive learning experiences. The integration of molecular biology, genetics, and computational biology into anatomical research has deepened the understanding of the body's structure and function at the cellular and molecular levels.

Basic Terminologies in Anatomy

Understanding the basic terminologies in anatomy is essential for anyone delving into the study of the human body. These terms not only provide a standard language for describing the locations and relationships of body parts but also facilitate clear communication among healthcare professionals, researchers, and students. This chapter will explore fundamental anatomical terms, helping beginners grasp the essential vocabulary needed to navigate the complex world of human anatomy.

Anatomy relies heavily on precise terminology to describe the human body's structures and their locations. Anatomical position is the reference point from which all anatomical terms are derived. In this standard position, the body is standing upright, facing forward, with arms at the sides and palms facing forward. Feet are flat on the ground and facing forward. This position ensures consistency in describing locations and directions on the body.

Directional terms are crucial for indicating the location of one body part relative to another. These terms are often paired to describe opposite directions. For instance, "superior" means above or toward the head, while "inferior" means below or toward the feet. Similarly, "anterior" (or "ventral") refers to the front of the body, and "posterior" (or "dorsal") refers to the back. "Medial" indicates a position closer to the midline of the body, whereas "lateral" means farther from the midline. "Proximal" and "distal" are terms used primarily for limbs; "proximal" means closer to the point of attachment to the body, and "distal" means farther from that point. Understanding these terms is fundamental for accurately describing the relative positions of structures within the body.

Anatomical planes are imaginary lines that divide the body into sections, providing reference points for studying the body's structures. The three primary planes are the sagittal, coronal, and transverse planes. The sagittal plane divides the body into left and right portions. If this division is exactly in the middle, it is called the midsagittal or median plane; if it is off to one side, it is referred to as a parasagittal plane. The coronal plane, also known as the frontal plane, divides the body into anterior (front) and posterior (back) portions. The transverse plane, or horizontal plane, divides the body into superior (upper) and inferior (lower) parts. These planes are essential for visualizing and describing locations in three-dimensional space.

Body cavities are another important aspect of anatomical terminology. These cavities are spaces within the body that house and protect internal organs. The two main cavities are the dorsal and ventral cavities. The dorsal cavity is subdivided into the cranial cavity, which encases the brain, and the spinal cavity, which encloses the spinal cord. The ventral cavity is larger and divided into the thoracic cavity and the abdominopelvic cavity. The thoracic cavity, located above the diaphragm, contains the heart and lungs. The abdominopelvic cavity, located below the diaphragm, is further divided into the abdominal cavity (housing digestive organs) and the pelvic cavity (containing the reproductive organs, bladder, and rectum).

Within these body cavities, specific terms describe the lining membranes. The serous membranes are thin tissues that line the body cavities and cover the organs within them. These membranes are divided into two layers: the parietal layer, which lines the cavity walls, and the visceral layer, which covers the organs. For instance, the pericardium is the serous membrane surrounding the heart, with the parietal pericardium lining the pericardial cavity and the visceral pericardium covering the heart itself. Similarly, the pleura is the serous membrane around the lungs, and the peritoneum surrounds the organs within the abdominopelvic cavity.

Regions of the body are another key component of anatomical terminology. The body is often divided into specific regions to facilitate study and communication. The axial region includes the head, neck, and trunk, while the appendicular region consists of the limbs. Each region can be further subdivided. For example, the trunk is divided into the thoracic (chest) region, the abdominal region, and the pelvic region. The upper limb includes the arm (brachium), forearm (antebrachium), wrist (carpus), and hand (manus), while the lower limb includes the thigh (femur), leg (crus), ankle (tarsus), and foot (pes). These regional terms help pinpoint specific areas and structures within the body.

Anatomical terms also describe the positions and movements of the body. Flexion and extension are movements that occur in the sagittal plane. Flexion decreases the angle between two body parts, such as bending the elbow, while extension increases the angle, such as straightening the elbow. Abduction and adduction occur in the coronal plane. Abduction moves a body part away from the midline, like lifting the arm to the side, while adduction moves it toward the midline. Rotation involves turning a body part around its axis, such as turning the head side to side. Other terms include elevation (lifting a body part upward), depression (moving it downward), pronation (rotating the forearm so the palm faces backward), and supination (rotating the forearm so the palm faces forward).

Understanding tissues and their classification is also fundamental in anatomy. Tissues are groups of similar cells that perform specific functions. There are four primary tissue types: epithelial, connective, muscle, and nervous tissues. Epithelial tissue covers body surfaces and lines cavities, providing protection, secretion, and absorption. Connective tissue supports and binds other tissues, with diverse types like bone, blood, and adipose tissue. Muscle tissue is responsible for movement, with three types: skeletal (voluntary movement), cardiac (heart contraction), and smooth (involuntary movement in organs). Nervous tissue transmits electrical impulses, coordinating bodily functions and responses.

The skeletal system is another critical area of anatomical terminology. Bones are classified by their shapes: long bones (like the femur), short bones (such as the carpals), flat bones (like the sternum), and irregular bones (such as the vertebrae). Each bone has specific landmarks and features. For instance, the humerus has a head, shaft, and condyles. Joints, where two or more bones meet, are classified by their structure and function. Synovial joints, like the knee, are freely movable, while fibrous joints, such as the sutures in the skull, are immovable. Understanding these terms is essential for studying the skeleton's structure and function.

The muscular system also uses specific terminology to describe muscles and their actions. Muscles are named based on various criteria: location (e.g., pectoralis major), shape (e.g., deltoid), size (e.g., gluteus maximus), direction of fibers (e.g., rectus abdominis), number of origins (e.g., biceps brachii), and action (e.g., extensor digitorum). Muscle actions are described using terms like agonist (primary mover), antagonist (opposes the primary mover), synergist (assists the primary mover), and fixator (stabilizes the origin of the primary mover).

The cardiovascular system includes terms related to the heart and blood vessels. The heart's anatomy includes the atria (upper chambers), ventricles (lower chambers), valves (such as the mitral and tricuspid valves), and major blood vessels (like the aorta and vena cava). Blood vessels are classified as arteries (carrying blood away from the heart), veins (carrying blood toward the heart), and capillaries (tiny vessels where exchange occurs between blood and tissues).

The nervous system's terminology encompasses the brain, spinal cord, and peripheral nerves. The brain is divided into regions like the cerebrum (responsible for higher functions), cerebellum (coordination and balance), and brainstem (basic life functions). The spinal cord is segmented into cervical, thoracic, lumbar, and sacral regions. Peripheral nerves are classified as cranial nerves (emerging from the brain) and spinal nerves (emerging from the spinal cord).

Levels of Structural Organization in the Human Body

The human body is an intricate structure composed of various levels of organization, each building upon the previous to form a complex, living organism. Understanding these levels of structural organization is crucial for comprehending how the body functions as a whole. By exploring these levels, we can appreciate the intricate design and functionality that enable us to perform daily activities, maintain homeostasis, and respond to environmental changes.

The simplest level of structural organization in the human body is the chemical level. At this level, atoms combine to form molecules. Atoms such as carbon, hydrogen, oxygen, and nitrogen are the fundamental building blocks of matter. These atoms come together to form molecules such as water, proteins, lipids, carbohydrates, and nucleic acids. These molecules are essential for various biochemical processes critical for life, including cellular respiration, protein synthesis, and DNA replication. For instance, the combination of oxygen and hydrogen atoms forms water, a molecule vital for most biochemical reactions within cells.

Next, the cellular level builds upon the chemical level. Cells are the basic structural and functional units of life. Each cell is composed of various molecules that work together to perform specific functions. Cells vary widely in size, shape, and function, reflecting their specialized roles within the body. For example, red blood cells are specialized for transporting oxygen, while nerve cells (neurons) are designed to transmit electrical impulses. Cells are surrounded by a plasma membrane, which regulates the movement of substances in and out of the cell. Inside the cell, organelles such as the nucleus, mitochondria, and endoplasmic reticulum perform distinct functions that contribute to the cell's overall activity.

Tissues are the next level of structural organization, formed by groups of similar cells working together to perform a common function. There are four primary types of tissues in the human body: epithelial, connective, muscle, and nervous tissues. Epithelial tissue covers body surfaces and lines cavities, providing protection, absorption, secretion, and sensation. Connective tissue supports, protects, and binds other tissues together; it includes bone, blood, adipose tissue, and cartilage. Muscle tissue is responsible for movement and consists of skeletal, cardiac, and smooth muscle types. Nervous tissue is involved in receiving, transmitting, and processing nerve impulses, and is composed of neurons and supporting glial cells.

Building upon tissues, the organ level of structural organization involves the combination of different tissue types to form organs. Each organ has a specific function and a unique structure that enables it to perform its role effectively. For example, the heart, composed of cardiac muscle tissue, connective tissue, and epithelial tissue, functions as a pump to circulate blood throughout the body. The stomach, comprising muscle tissue, epithelial tissue, and connective tissue, plays a crucial role in the digestion of food. Other examples of organs include the lungs, liver, kidneys, and brain. Each organ's structure is intricately related to its function, demonstrating the principle that form follows function.

The organ system level involves groups of organs that work together to perform complex functions necessary for the body's survival and well-being. There are 11 major organ systems in the human body: the integumentary, skeletal, muscular, nervous, endocrine, cardiovascular, lymphatic, respiratory, digestive, urinary, and reproductive systems. Each system has distinct but interrelated roles. For example, the cardiovascular system, comprising the heart and blood vessels, transports nutrients, oxygen, and waste products throughout the body. The respiratory system, including the lungs and airways, facilitates gas exchange, supplying oxygen to the blood and removing carbon dioxide. The digestive system, consisting of organs such as the stomach, intestines, and liver, breaks down food, absorbs nutrients, and eliminates waste. These systems do not operate in isolation; they work in concert to maintain homeostasis, the body's stable internal environment.

Finally, the organismal level is the highest level of structural organization. At this level, all the organ systems come together to form a complete living organism—the human body. The integration and coordination of all organ systems enable the body to function as a unified whole. This level of organization allows for complex behaviors, adaptation to environmental changes, reproduction, and survival. For instance, when you engage in physical activity, multiple organ systems, including the muscular, respiratory, cardiovascular, and nervous systems, work together to ensure adequate oxygen delivery, energy production, and waste removal.

Understanding the levels of structural organization in the human body provides a framework for studying anatomy and physiology. It highlights the interdependence of all biological structures and functions, from the smallest chemical components to the entire organism. This hierarchical organization ensures that the body operates efficiently and effectively, adapting to various demands and maintaining homeostasis.

One practical application of this knowledge is in the field of medicine. Medical practitioners use their understanding of these levels to diagnose and treat illnesses. For instance, a disease might originate at the cellular level, such as cancer, where abnormal cells proliferate uncontrollably. Treatment may target these cells specifically, using chemotherapy or radiation. Similarly, understanding the tissue and organ levels can help in surgical procedures, where precise knowledge of tissue structures and organ locations is crucial.

Another example is in sports science, where understanding the muscular and skeletal systems helps in designing training programs that enhance performance and prevent injury. Knowledge of the cardiovascular and respiratory systems is essential for developing effective cardiovascular training regimens.

In education, teaching the levels of structural organization helps students build a solid foundation in biology. By learning how atoms and molecules form cells, how cells form tissues, and how tissues form organs and organ systems, students can appreciate the complexity and interconnectedness of the human body. This foundational knowledge is crucial for advanced studies in health, medicine, and biological sciences.

Homeostasis and Its Significance

Homeostasis is a fundamental concept in biology that refers to the ability of an organism to maintain a stable internal environment despite changes in external conditions. This dynamic equilibrium is crucial for the survival and optimal functioning of living organisms. The term "homeostasis" was coined by Walter Bradford Cannon in the early 20th century, building on the earlier work of Claude Bernard, who introduced the idea of the "internal environment." The significance of homeostasis cannot be overstated, as it underpins the stability necessary for biological processes to occur efficiently.

The human body has evolved intricate mechanisms to regulate various physiological parameters, ensuring they remain within narrow limits. Key aspects of homeostasis include the regulation of temperature, pH, glucose levels, and electrolyte balance. Each of these parameters is tightly controlled by feedback systems that involve sensors, control centers, and effectors working in harmony.

Temperature regulation is one of the most critical aspects of homeostasis. The human body maintains a core temperature of approximately 37°C (98.6°F). This temperature is optimal for enzymatic reactions and metabolic processes. The hypothalamus, a region of the brain, acts as the body's thermostat. When body temperature deviates from the set point, the hypothalamus triggers responses to restore balance. For example, in response to overheating, the body initiates sweating and vasodilation (widening of blood vessels) to dissipate heat. Conversely, in response to cold, the body induces shivering and vasoconstriction (narrowing of blood vessels) to conserve heat.

pH regulation is another vital component of homeostasis. The body's pH is maintained around 7.4, which is slightly alkaline. This balance is crucial for the proper functioning of enzymes and cellular processes. The bicarbonate buffer system, respiratory system, and renal system work together to regulate pH. The bicarbonate buffer system neutralizes excess acids or bases in the blood. The respiratory system adjusts the exhalation of carbon dioxide, which can affect blood pH. The kidneys excrete or retain hydrogen and bicarbonate ions to fine-tune pH levels.

Glucose regulation ensures that cells receive a steady supply of energy while preventing the harmful effects of excessive glucose. The pancreas plays a pivotal role in this process by secreting insulin and glucagon. When blood glucose levels rise after a meal, the pancreas releases insulin, which facilitates the uptake of glucose by cells and its storage as glycogen in the liver. When blood glucose levels drop, the pancreas releases glucagon, which stimulates the breakdown of glycogen into glucose. This balance prevents hyperglycemia (high blood sugar) and hypoglycemia (low blood sugar).

Electrolyte balance is essential for nerve function, muscle contraction, and fluid balance. Key electrolytes include sodium, potassium, calcium, and chloride. The kidneys regulate electrolyte levels by filtering the blood and excreting excess ions through urine. Hormones such as aldosterone and antidiuretic hormone (ADH) play crucial roles in this regulation. Aldosterone increases sodium reabsorption and potassium excretion, while ADH promotes water reabsorption to maintain fluid balance.

The concept of negative feedback is central to homeostasis. Negative feedback mechanisms counteract deviations from a set point, restoring balance. For instance, in temperature regulation, an increase in body temperature triggers mechanisms to cool the body, while a decrease in temperature triggers mechanisms to warm the body. This feedback loop ensures that physiological parameters remain within their optimal range.

Positive feedback mechanisms, although less common, also play a role in certain physiological processes. Unlike negative feedback, positive feedback amplifies a response until a specific outcome is achieved. A classic example is the process of childbirth. The release of oxytocin during labor intensifies uterine contractions, which in turn stimulate more oxytocin release. This cycle continues until the baby is born. While positive feedback is not typically involved in maintaining homeostasis, it is crucial for specific functions that require a rapid and decisive response.

Disruptions to homeostasis can lead to various health issues. For example, failure in temperature regulation can result in hyperthermia or hypothermia, both of which can be life-threatening. Imbalances in blood pH can lead to acidosis or alkalosis, conditions that can severely impact cellular function. Dysregulation of glucose levels is associated with diabetes mellitus, a chronic condition that can cause significant complications if not managed properly. Electrolyte imbalances can affect heart rhythm, muscle function, and neurological activity.

The body's ability to maintain homeostasis is influenced by various factors, including age, genetics, lifestyle, and environmental conditions. As individuals age, the efficiency of homeostatic mechanisms can decline, making them more susceptible to health issues. Genetic factors can predispose individuals to certain conditions that affect homeostasis, such as diabetes or hypertension.

Lifestyle choices, including diet, exercise, and stress management, play a significant role in supporting or undermining homeostatic balance. Environmental factors, such as temperature and altitude, can also challenge the body's homeostatic mechanisms.

Understanding homeostasis provides valuable insights into health and disease. For healthcare professionals, monitoring and supporting homeostatic mechanisms is a key aspect of patient care. For example, managing a diabetic patient involves regular monitoring of blood glucose levels and adjusting insulin therapy to maintain glucose homeostasis. In critical care settings, maintaining electrolyte balance, pH, and temperature are vital for patient survival.

Preventive measures can help support homeostasis and overall health. A balanced diet that provides essential nutrients supports metabolic processes and energy balance. Regular physical activity enhances cardiovascular and respiratory function, aiding in the regulation of glucose and lipid levels. Adequate hydration is crucial for maintaining electrolyte balance and kidney function. Stress management techniques, such as mindfulness and relaxation exercises, can mitigate the negative impact of chronic stress on homeostatic mechanisms.

The interplay between different organ systems highlights the complexity of homeostasis. For instance, during exercise, the cardiovascular, respiratory, and muscular systems work together to meet the increased demand for oxygen and nutrients. The cardiovascular system increases heart rate and blood flow to muscles, the respiratory system enhances oxygen intake and carbon dioxide expulsion, and the muscular system utilizes the oxygen and nutrients for energy production. This coordinated response ensures that the body can perform physical activity efficiently while maintaining internal balance.

Chapter 2

The Cellular Basis of Life

Overview of Cell Structure and Function

Cells are the fundamental building blocks of all living organisms. Understanding their structure and function is crucial to grasping the complexities of biology. At the core of this understanding is the realization that while cells can vary significantly in size, shape, and function, they share common structural features that facilitate their roles in sustaining life.

The cell membrane, also known as the plasma membrane, is a critical component of all cells. This semi-permeable membrane encloses the cell, providing it with structural support and regulating the movement of substances in and out of the cell. The membrane is composed of a phospholipid bilayer with embedded proteins, cholesterol, and carbohydrates. The fluid mosaic model describes this structure, highlighting the dynamic nature of the membrane, where lipids and proteins can move laterally within the layer.

Within the cell membrane lies the cytoplasm, a jelly-like substance that houses various organelles and is the site of numerous metabolic reactions. The cytoplasm is composed primarily of water, salts, and organic molecules, providing a medium for biochemical processes and acting as a buffer to protect cellular components.

One of the most prominent organelles within eukaryotic cells is the nucleus. The nucleus serves as the control center of the cell, housing the cell's genetic material in the form of DNA. The nuclear envelope, a double membrane, surrounds the nucleus, with nuclear pores allowing the selective exchange of materials between the nucleus and the cytoplasm. Within the nucleus, the nucleolus is responsible for ribosomal RNA (rRNA) synthesis and ribosome assembly.

Ribosomes, either free-floating in the cytoplasm or attached to the endoplasmic reticulum (ER), are the sites of protein synthesis. The endoplasmic reticulum is categorized into two types: rough ER, which has ribosomes attached to its surface and is involved in protein synthesis and modification, and smooth ER, which lacks ribosomes and is involved in lipid synthesis and detoxification processes.

The Golgi apparatus, another vital organelle, functions as the cell's packaging and distribution center. It modifies, sorts, and packages proteins and lipids received from the ER for transport to their destined locations within or outside the cell. The Golgi apparatus is composed of flattened membrane-bound sacs called cisternae, where the processing and sorting of macromolecules occur.

Mitochondria, often referred to as the powerhouses of the cell, generate the energy required for various cellular activities. These organelles convert energy stored in organic molecules into adenosine triphosphate (ATP) through cellular respiration. Mitochondria have a double membrane, with the inner membrane folding into cristae to increase surface area for energy production. Interestingly, mitochondria contain their own DNA and ribosomes, suggesting an evolutionary origin from ancient symbiotic bacteria.

Plant cells contain some unique organelles not found in animal cells, such as chloroplasts and a central vacuole. Chloroplasts are the sites of photosynthesis, where light energy is converted into chemical energy stored in glucose. These organelles contain chlorophyll, the pigment responsible for capturing light energy. Like mitochondria, chloroplasts have their own DNA and are believed to have originated from symbiotic bacteria. The central vacuole, a large membrane-bound compartment, serves multiple functions, including storage of nutrients and waste products, maintenance of turgor pressure, and degradation of complex molecules.

Lysosomes and peroxisomes are specialized organelles involved in the breakdown and recycling of cellular materials. Lysosomes contain hydrolytic enzymes that digest macromolecules, damaged organelles, and pathogens. Peroxisomes carry out oxidation reactions that detoxify harmful substances and break down fatty acids. Both organelles play crucial roles in maintaining cellular homeostasis and protecting the cell from damage.

The cytoskeleton, an intricate network of protein fibers, provides structural support and facilitates cell movement, shape changes, and intracellular transport. The cytoskeleton is composed of microfilaments, intermediate filaments, and microtubules. Microfilaments, made of actin, are involved in cell movement and muscle contraction. Intermediate filaments provide mechanical strength to cells and help maintain their shape. Microtubules, composed of tubulin, form the spindle fibers during cell division and serve as tracks for the movement of organelles and vesicles within the cell.

Cellular communication is essential for coordinating the activities of multicellular organisms. Cells communicate through direct contact, chemical signals, and electrical signals. Gap junctions and plasmodesmata are specialized structures that allow direct communication between adjacent cells. Gap junctions, found in animal cells, are channels that enable the exchange of ions and small molecules. Plasmodesmata, found in plant cells, are cytoplasmic channels that traverse the cell walls, allowing the transport of molecules and communication between cells.

Chemical signaling involves the release of signaling molecules, such as hormones and neurotransmitters, which bind to specific receptors on target cells, triggering a response. This process can be classified into autocrine signaling (where cells respond to signals they produce), paracrine signaling (where signals affect neighboring cells), and endocrine signaling (where signals travel through the bloodstream to distant cells).

Electrical signaling is crucial in the nervous system, where neurons transmit signals in the form of action potentials. These electrical impulses travel along the axon of a neuron and trigger the release of neurotransmitters at synapses, facilitating communication with other neurons, muscles, or glands.

Understanding cell structure and function also extends to the cell cycle and cell division. The cell cycle consists of interphase and the mitotic phase. During interphase, the cell grows, replicates its DNA, and prepares for division. The mitotic phase includes mitosis, where the duplicated chromosomes are separated into two daughter nuclei, and cytokinesis, where the cytoplasm is divided, resulting in two genetically identical daughter cells.

Mitosis is a tightly regulated process consisting of several stages: prophase, metaphase, anaphase, and telophase. During prophase, chromatin condenses into visible chromosomes, and the nuclear envelope breaks down. In metaphase, chromosomes align at the cell's equatorial plane. Anaphase involves the separation of sister chromatids to opposite poles of the cell. Finally, during telophase, the nuclear envelope re-forms around the separated chromosomes, and the cell prepares to divide its cytoplasm.

In contrast to mitosis, meiosis is a type of cell division that reduces the chromosome number by half, resulting in four genetically diverse haploid cells. This process is essential for sexual reproduction and involves two consecutive divisions: meiosis I and meiosis II. Meiosis introduces genetic variation through mechanisms such as crossing over and independent assortment of chromosomes.

The study of cell structure and function is not limited to eukaryotic cells; prokaryotic cells, such as bacteria, also play vital roles in ecosystems and human health. Prokaryotic cells lack a nucleus and membrane-bound organelles, but they possess essential structures such as the cell wall, plasma membrane, cytoplasm, ribosomes, and genetic material located in the nucleoid region.

Prokaryotic cells exhibit diverse shapes and arrangements, including cocci (spherical), bacilli (rod-shaped), and spirilla (spiral-shaped). They can form colonies, biofilms, or exist as single cells. Prokaryotes reproduce asexually through binary fission, a process where a single cell divides into two identical daughter cells.

Cell Membrane and Transport Mechanisms

Imagine a bustling city with gates, checkpoints, and highways, each meticulously regulating the flow of people and goods. This city, in many ways, mirrors the intricate workings of a cell, particularly its cell membrane, which serves as both a guardian and a facilitator. The cell membrane's primary function is to maintain homeostasis by controlling the entry and exit of various substances. This dynamic barrier is composed of a phospholipid bilayer interspersed with proteins, cholesterol, and carbohydrates, each contributing to its fluidity and functionality.

The phospholipid bilayer forms the fundamental structure of the cell membrane. Phospholipids are unique molecules with hydrophilic (water-attracting) heads and hydrophobic (water-repelling) tails. When these molecules align, they create a double-layered membrane with the hydrophobic tails facing inward, shielded from water, while the hydrophilic heads face outward. This arrangement not only provides a stable barrier but also allows the membrane to be fluid and flexible, essential for various cellular processes.

Embedded within this bilayer are proteins that perform a myriad of functions. Integral proteins span the entire membrane, acting as channels or transporters to facilitate the movement of substances that cannot pass through the lipid bilayer on their own. Peripheral proteins, on the other hand, are attached to the exterior or interior surfaces of the membrane and play roles in signaling and maintaining the cell's shape. These proteins, along with cholesterol molecules interspersed within the bilayer, contribute to the membrane's stability and fluidity, ensuring it remains functional under various conditions.

Transport across the cell membrane can occur via passive or active mechanisms. Passive transport does not require energy and relies on the concentration gradient, the difference in the concentration of a substance across a space. This gradient drives the movement of substances from areas of higher concentration to areas of lower concentration. There are three main types of passive transport: simple diffusion, facilitated diffusion, and osmosis.

Simple diffusion involves the movement of small, nonpolar molecules, such as oxygen and carbon dioxide, directly through the phospholipid bilayer. As these molecules move down their concentration gradient, they pass freely across the membrane without the aid of transport proteins. This process is crucial for respiratory gas exchange in cells.

Facilitated diffusion, however, requires the assistance of transport proteins to move substances across the membrane. Channel proteins form pores that allow specific molecules or ions to pass through, while carrier proteins undergo conformational changes to transport their cargo. For example, glucose, a polar molecule, relies on carrier proteins to enter cells, ensuring it reaches the interior where it can be used for energy production.

Osmosis is a specialized form of passive transport that involves the movement of water molecules across a selectively permeable membrane. Water moves from an area of lower solute concentration (higher water concentration) to an area of higher solute concentration (lower water concentration) until equilibrium is reached. This process is vital for maintaining cell turgor in plants and the overall fluid balance in animal cells.

Active transport mechanisms, in contrast, require energy in the form of adenosine triphosphate (ATP) to move substances against their concentration gradient, from areas of lower concentration to areas of higher concentration. Primary active transport directly uses ATP to fuel the transport process. The sodium-potassium pump, a well-known example, moves three sodium ions out of the cell and two potassium ions into the cell, maintaining essential electrochemical gradients crucial for nerve impulse transmission and muscle contraction.

Secondary active transport, or cotransport, uses the energy stored in the form of an electrochemical gradient created by primary active transport. In this mechanism, one substance moves down its gradient, providing the energy to transport another substance against its gradient. Symporters and antiporters are the two types of cotransporters: symporters move substances in the same direction, while antiporters move them in opposite directions. The sodium-glucose cotransporter in the intestines, for instance, uses the sodium gradient established by the sodium-potassium pump to bring glucose into cells against its gradient.

In addition to these transport mechanisms, cells employ vesicular transport to move large molecules or particles across the membrane. This process involves the formation of vesicles, small membrane-bound sacs that can encapsulate substances for transport. Endocytosis and exocytosis are the two main types of vesicular transport.

Endocytosis allows cells to engulf external substances by enclosing them in a vesicle formed from the cell membrane. There are three forms of endocytosis: phagocytosis, pinocytosis, and receptor-mediated endocytosis. Phagocytosis, or "cell eating," involves the engulfment of large particles or even other cells, such as how white blood cells ingest pathogens. Pinocytosis, or "cell drinking," involves the ingestion of extracellular fluid and its dissolved solutes. Receptor-mediated endocytosis is a more selective process where specific molecules bind to receptors on the cell surface, triggering vesicle formation to internalize the bound substances.

Exocytosis is the reverse process, where substances contained in vesicles are expelled from the cell. This mechanism is crucial for the secretion of various molecules, such as hormones, neurotransmitters, and digestive enzymes. The vesicle membrane fuses with the cell membrane, releasing its contents into the extracellular space.

The intricate dance of molecules across the cell membrane is not only fascinating but also critical for life. Understanding these transport mechanisms provides insight into how cells interact with their environment, obtain nutrients, expel waste, and communicate with other cells. This knowledge has profound implications for medicine and biotechnology. For example, targeting specific transport proteins can influence drug delivery and the treatment of diseases. Cystic fibrosis, a genetic disorder, is caused by mutations in the CFTR protein, a chloride channel, leading to impaired ion transport and mucus buildup in the lungs. By studying and manipulating these transport pathways, researchers can develop therapies to alleviate such conditions.

Moreover, the principles of cell membrane transport are harnessed in various biotechnological applications. Liposomes, artificial vesicles, are used to deliver drugs and genetic material to specific cells, enhancing the precision and efficacy of treatments. Understanding osmosis and diffusion is also critical in the design of dialysis machines, which filter waste products from the blood of patients with kidney failure.

In agricultural biotechnology, manipulating transport mechanisms in plant cells can improve nutrient uptake and resistance to environmental stressors. For instance, enhancing the expression of specific transporters can increase a plant's ability to absorb essential minerals from the soil, promoting better growth and yield.

Cellular Metabolism and Energy Production

Life at its core is a series of chemical reactions, orchestrated with precision to sustain the intricate processes of living organisms. Central to this symphony is cellular metabolism, the set of biochemical reactions that occur within a cell to maintain life. These reactions are broadly classified into two categories: catabolic pathways that break down molecules to produce energy and anabolic pathways that use energy to build complex molecules. To truly understand how cells harness and utilize energy, we delve into the processes of cellular respiration and photosynthesis, both of which illustrate the remarkable efficiency and adaptability of living systems.

The journey of energy production in cells typically begins with glucose, a simple sugar that serves as a primary energy source. The process of extracting energy from glucose involves glycolysis, the citric acid cycle (Krebs cycle), and oxidative phosphorylation, which together constitute cellular respiration. Glycolysis, the first step, occurs in the cytoplasm and does not require oxygen. During glycolysis, one molecule of glucose is broken down into two molecules of pyruvate, yielding a small amount of energy in the form of two ATP molecules and two NADH molecules.

The fate of pyruvate depends on the presence of oxygen. In aerobic conditions, pyruvate enters the mitochondria, where it is converted into acetyl-CoA, a crucial substrate for the citric acid cycle. This cycle, taking place in the mitochondrial matrix, systematically oxidizes acetyl-CoA, producing carbon dioxide as a waste product and transferring high-energy electrons to NADH and $FADH_2$. These electron carriers then shuttle their high-energy electrons to the electron transport chain, a series of protein complexes embedded in the inner mitochondrial membrane.

The electron transport chain is where the magic of oxidative phosphorylation happens. As electrons pass through these complexes, they release energy, which is used to pump protons across the inner mitochondrial membrane, creating an electrochemical gradient. This gradient drives the synthesis of ATP by ATP synthase, a process known as chemiosmosis. The culmination of this electron transfer is the reduction of oxygen to water, underscoring the critical role of oxygen in aerobic respiration. Through these stages, a single molecule of glucose can yield up to 36-38 ATP molecules, highlighting the efficiency of cellular respiration.

However, in the absence of oxygen, cells can resort to anaerobic respiration or fermentation to meet their energy needs. In muscle cells, for example, pyruvate is reduced to lactate, which can accumulate during intense exercise, leading to the familiar sensation of muscle fatigue. Yeast cells, on the other hand, convert pyruvate to ethanol and carbon dioxide, a process exploited in brewing and baking industries.

While cellular respiration is essential for animal cells, plant cells have an additional trick up their sleeve: photosynthesis. This process allows plants to convert light energy into chemical energy, stored in the bonds of glucose. Photosynthesis occurs in chloroplasts, organelles equipped with pigments such as chlorophyll that capture light energy. The process can be divided into two stages: the light-dependent reactions and the Calvin cycle.

During the light-dependent reactions, which take place in the thylakoid membranes, chlorophyll absorbs light energy, exciting electrons to a higher energy state. These high-energy electrons are then transferred through an electron transport chain, similar to that in mitochondria, resulting in the production of ATP and NADPH. Water molecules are split to replace the lost electrons, releasing oxygen as a byproduct.

The ATP and NADPH generated in the light-dependent reactions are then used in the Calvin cycle, which occurs in the stroma of the chloroplasts. Here, carbon dioxide is fixed into a stable intermediate and eventually converted into glucose through a series of enzyme-driven reactions. This glucose can then be used by the plant for energy or serve as a building block for more complex carbohydrates like starch and cellulose.

Understanding the dual processes of cellular respiration and photosynthesis provides a comprehensive picture of how cells manage energy.

These pathways are not isolated but interlinked in a global cycle of energy transfer. The oxygen produced during photosynthesis is essential for aerobic respiration, while the carbon dioxide released during respiration is a key substrate for photosynthesis. This elegant balance sustains life on Earth, showcasing the interdependence of different organisms and their metabolic pathways.

On a cellular level, the regulation of these metabolic pathways is crucial for maintaining homeostasis. Cells must constantly adjust their metabolic rates in response to internal and external signals. Hormones such as insulin and glucagon play a critical role in this regulation. Insulin promotes the uptake and storage of glucose, lowering blood sugar levels, while glucagon triggers the release of glucose from stored glycogen, raising blood sugar levels. Additionally, the availability of substrates, presence of inhibitors, and feedback mechanisms ensure that metabolic pathways operate efficiently and adaptively.

Modern research into cellular metabolism has far-reaching implications, from understanding disease mechanisms to developing novel therapies. For instance, cancer cells often exhibit altered metabolic pathways, known as the Warburg effect, where they preferentially use glycolysis even in the presence of oxygen. This metabolic reprogramming supports rapid cell division and growth, providing potential targets for cancer treatment.

Moreover, advancements in biotechnology harness the principles of cellular metabolism for various applications. Bioengineers are developing microorganisms capable of producing biofuels, pharmaceuticals, and other valuable compounds through metabolic engineering. By manipulating metabolic pathways, scientists aim to create more efficient and sustainable production methods.

In the realm of medicine, metabolic disorders such as diabetes highlight the importance of understanding and managing cellular metabolism. Diabetes results from the body's inability to regulate blood sugar levels properly, either due to insufficient insulin production or insulin resistance. Treatments often focus on restoring metabolic balance through medication, diet, and lifestyle changes.

Cell Division: Mitosis and Meiosis

Cell division is a fundamental process that enables organisms to grow, develop, and reproduce. It is through cell division that life perpetuates itself, ensuring that genetic information is accurately passed from one generation to the next. There are two primary types of cell division: mitosis and meiosis. Both processes are essential but serve different purposes and occur through distinct mechanisms. Understanding these processes provides insight into the continuity of life, the complexity of development, and the genetic diversity that is crucial for evolution.

Mitosis is the process by which a single cell divides to produce two genetically identical daughter cells. It is the means by which somatic cells—those that make up the body tissues—are produced. Mitosis ensures that each daughter cell receives a complete set of chromosomes, maintaining the diploid number characteristic of the species. The process of mitosis is divided into several phases: prophase, metaphase, anaphase, and telophase, followed by cytokinesis.

During prophase, the chromatin condenses into visible chromosomes, each consisting of two sister chromatids joined at the centromere. The nuclear envelope begins to disintegrate, and the spindle apparatus starts to form. The centrosomes, which have replicated during the previous interphase, move to opposite poles of the cell, organizing the microtubules that will facilitate chromosome movement.

Metaphase is characterized by the alignment of the chromosomes along the metaphase plate, an imaginary plane equidistant from the two spindle poles. The spindle fibers attach to the centromeres of the chromosomes, ensuring that each sister chromatid will be pulled to opposite poles of the cell.

Anaphase follows as the shortest phase, where the centromeres split, and the sister chromatids are pulled apart by the spindle fibers toward opposite poles. This separation ensures that each daughter cell will receive an identical set of chromosomes.

During telophase, the chromatids reach the poles, and the nuclear envelope re-forms around each set of chromosomes, which begin to decondense back into chromatin. The spindle apparatus disassembles, and the cell prepares to divide its cytoplasm.

Cytokinesis, the final step, involves the division of the cytoplasm and the formation of two distinct daughter cells. In animal cells, a contractile ring of actin filaments pinches the cell membrane inward, creating a cleavage furrow that eventually splits the cell in two. In plant cells, a cell plate forms along the line of division, eventually developing into a separating wall.

Meiosis, on the other hand, is the process by which gametes—sperm and eggs—are produced. It consists of two sequential divisions, meiosis I and meiosis II, resulting in four non-identical haploid cells, each with half the number of chromosomes of the original cell. Meiosis introduces genetic diversity through mechanisms such as crossing over and independent assortment.

Meiosis I begins with prophase I, where homologous chromosomes pair up in a process called synapsis, forming tetrads. This close pairing allows for crossing over, where homologous chromosomes exchange genetic material, creating new combinations of alleles. This genetic recombination is a crucial source of genetic diversity.

In metaphase I, the tetrads align on the metaphase plate, with spindle fibers from opposite poles attaching to each homologous chromosome. This arrangement ensures that when the homologous chromosomes separate during anaphase I, each daughter cell will receive a mix of maternal and paternal chromosomes.

Telophase I and cytokinesis result in two haploid cells, each with half the original number of chromosomes, but each chromosome still consists of two sister chromatids.

Meiosis II resembles a mitotic division. During prophase II, the chromosomes condense again, and the spindle apparatus forms in each haploid cell. In metaphase II, the chromosomes align along the metaphase plate, and in anaphase II, the sister chromatids are finally separated and pulled to opposite poles. Telophase II and cytokinesis complete the process, resulting in four haploid daughter cells, each genetically distinct from one another and from the original parent cell.

The significance of meiosis extends beyond just the production of gametes. By reducing the chromosome number by half, meiosis ensures that when fertilization occurs, the resulting zygote has the correct diploid number. The genetic variation introduced by crossing over and independent assortment during meiosis is vital for evolution, as it provides a population with a diverse genetic pool from which natural selection can act.

Errors in cell division, particularly during meiosis, can lead to significant consequences. Nondisjunction, where chromosomes fail to separate properly, can result in aneuploidy, a condition where cells have an abnormal number of chromosomes. This can lead to disorders such as Down syndrome, where individuals have an extra copy of chromosome 21, or Turner syndrome, where females have only one X chromosome.

Understanding cell division is not only fundamental to biology but also to medicine and agriculture. For example, cancer is characterized by uncontrolled cell division, often due to mutations in genes that regulate the cell cycle. Research into the mechanisms of mitosis and meiosis can lead to better cancer treatments by targeting specific stages of cell division.

In agriculture, manipulating meiosis in plants can help produce crops with desirable traits, such as disease resistance or increased yield.

To visualize these complex processes, imagine a choreographed dance. Each chromosome, spindle fiber, and cellular structure moves with precision, guided by an intricate set of signals and checkpoints. Just as a dance requires practice and coordination, cell division relies on a highly regulated sequence of events, ensuring that each step is executed correctly.

In the broader context of life, cell division is a testament to the elegance and efficiency of biological systems. From the single-cell zygote that divides and differentiates to form a complex organism, to the production of gametes that ensure the continuity of species, cell division is at the heart of life's perpetuation. It illustrates the balance between stability and change, where the faithful replication of genetic material coexists with the introduction of genetic diversity, driving evolution and adaptation.

Specialized Cells and Their Functions

Specialized cells are the cornerstone of multicellular organisms, each uniquely adapted to perform specific functions essential for survival. This differentiation allows organisms to carry out complex tasks through a division of labor, where different cell types contribute to the overall function and health of the body. From the oxygen-transporting red blood cells to the signal-transmitting neurons, specialized cells exemplify the remarkable adaptability and efficiency of biological systems.

Red blood cells (RBCs) are perhaps the most well-known specialized cells, crucial for oxygen transport. These cells are biconcave disks, a shape that increases their surface area for oxygen absorption and allows them to easily navigate through the narrowest capillaries. Lacking a nucleus and most organelles, RBCs are packed with hemoglobin, the protein responsible for binding and transporting oxygen from the lungs to tissues throughout the body and returning carbon dioxide to the lungs for exhalation. This specialization is vital for maintaining the body's oxygen levels and facilitating cellular respiration, the process by which cells generate energy.

Neurons, another example of specialized cells, form the foundation of the nervous system. Designed for rapid communication, neurons transmit electrical and chemical signals between different parts of the body. Each neuron consists of a cell body, dendrites, and an axon. The dendrites receive incoming signals, which are processed in the cell body and transmitted along the axon to other neurons or muscles. Myelin, a fatty substance that insulates the axon, speeds up signal transmission, ensuring that messages are conveyed quickly and efficiently. This rapid communication is essential for coordinating complex movements, processing sensory information, and regulating behavior and cognition.

Muscle cells, or myocytes, are specialized for contraction and movement. There are three types of muscle cells: skeletal, cardiac, and smooth. Skeletal muscle cells are long, cylindrical, and multinucleated, designed for voluntary movements and capable of powerful contractions. Cardiac muscle cells, found in the heart, are branched and interconnected, enabling synchronized contractions that pump blood throughout the body. Smooth muscle cells, located in the walls of internal organs, are spindle-shaped and control involuntary movements such as peristalsis in the digestive tract. The unique structures and functions of these muscle cells reflect their specialized roles in movement and force generation.

Epithelial cells line the surfaces of organs and structures throughout the body, forming protective barriers and facilitating absorption and secretion. These cells are tightly packed and can vary in shape—from thin, flat squamous cells to columnar cells. For example, the epithelial cells lining the intestines are specialized for nutrient absorption, featuring microvilli that increase surface area. In contrast, epithelial cells in the skin form a protective barrier against pathogens and physical damage. The specialization of epithelial cells is crucial for maintaining the integrity and function of organs and tissues.

White blood cells (WBCs), or leukocytes, are specialized cells of the immune system, designed to protect the body against infections and foreign invaders. There are several types of white blood cells, each with unique functions. Neutrophils are the first responders to infection sites, engulfing and destroying pathogens through phagocytosis. Lymphocytes, which include B cells and T cells, are central to the adaptive immune response. B cells produce antibodies that target specific antigens, while T cells destroy infected cells and coordinate the immune response. The diversity and specialization of white blood cells enable the immune system to respond effectively to a wide range of threats.

Adipocytes, or fat cells, are specialized for energy storage and insulation. These cells store triglycerides, which can be broken down into fatty acids and glycerol when energy is needed. Adipocytes also play a role in regulating metabolism and hormone production. For instance, they release leptin, a hormone that helps regulate appetite and energy balance. The ability of adipocytes to store and release energy as needed is essential for maintaining energy homeostasis in the body.

Osteocytes, the primary cells in bone tissue, are specialized for maintaining bone structure and function. These cells originate from osteoblasts, which secrete the extracellular matrix that forms bone. Once embedded in the matrix, osteoblasts become osteocytes, which extend long, branching processes that communicate with other bone cells and help regulate mineral content. This specialization allows osteocytes to play a critical role in bone remodeling and repair, ensuring the skeleton remains strong and resilient.

Sperm and egg cells, or gametes, are specialized for reproduction. Sperm cells are streamlined for mobility, with a flagellum that propels them toward the egg. They carry genetic material in the form of DNA and are equipped with enzymes to penetrate the egg's outer layers. Egg cells, in contrast, are large and nutrient-rich, providing the necessary resources for the developing embryo. The specialization of these gametes ensures successful fertilization and the continuation of genetic information to the next generation.

Stem cells are unique among specialized cells due to their potential to differentiate into various cell types. Embryonic stem cells can give rise to any cell type in the body, making them pluripotent. Adult stem cells, found in tissues like bone marrow and the brain, are more limited in their differentiation potential but are crucial for tissue repair and regeneration. The ability of stem cells to generate specialized cells is a focal point of regenerative medicine, offering potential treatments for a variety of conditions, from spinal cord injuries to degenerative diseases.

The specialization of cells extends beyond their individual structures and functions, contributing to the overall organization and efficiency of the body. In tissues and organs, different cell types work together in harmony, creating complex systems that perform vital functions. For example, in the digestive system, specialized cells in the stomach produce acid and enzymes to break down food, while cells in the intestines absorb nutrients. In the circulatory system, heart muscle cells pump blood, while endothelial cells line blood vessels, ensuring smooth blood flow and nutrient delivery.

The specialization of cells is a testament to the evolutionary processes that have shaped life on Earth. Each cell type has evolved unique structures and functions that enable it to perform specific tasks efficiently. This specialization allows multicellular organisms to adapt to their environments and survive in diverse conditions. The study of specialized cells not only enhances our understanding of biology but also informs medical and scientific advancements, leading to improved health outcomes and innovative therapies.

Chapter 3

Tissues: The Fabric of the Body

Classification of Tissues

Tissues are groups of cells that work together to perform specific functions. The classification of tissues is a fundamental concept in biology and medicine, providing a framework for understanding how the body is organized and functions. Tissues are broadly classified into four main types: epithelial, connective, muscle, and nervous tissues. Each type has distinct characteristics and functions, reflecting the diverse roles they play in the body.

Epithelial tissue covers body surfaces, lines cavities, and forms glands. It serves as a protective barrier, regulates the exchange of substances, and provides sensory functions. Epithelial cells are tightly packed, with minimal extracellular material, and they exhibit polarity, meaning they have an apical surface facing the body surface or cavity and a basal surface attached to underlying connective tissue. This arrangement allows epithelial tissue to protect underlying structures and control the movement of substances.

There are several types of epithelial tissues, categorized based on the shape of the cells and the number of cell layers. Simple epithelium consists of a single layer of cells, while stratified epithelium has multiple layers. For example, simple squamous epithelium, with its flat, thin cells, is ideal for diffusion and filtration, making it essential in the alveoli of the lungs and the glomeruli of the kidneys. Simple cuboidal epithelium, composed of cube-shaped cells, is found in glands and ducts, where it functions in secretion and absorption. Simple columnar epithelium, with tall, column-like cells, lines the digestive tract and is specialized for absorption and secretion. Stratified squamous epithelium, with multiple layers of flat cells, provides robust protection against abrasion and is found in the skin, mouth, and esophagus.

Connective tissue supports, binds, and protects other tissues and organs. It is characterized by an abundant extracellular matrix, which can be fluid, gelatinous, or solid, depending on the type of connective tissue. This matrix, composed of protein fibers like collagen and elastin, and ground substance, provides structural support and mediates the exchange of nutrients and waste between tissues and the bloodstream.

Connective tissues are diverse and include loose connective tissue, dense connective tissue, cartilage, bone, and blood. Loose connective tissue, such as areolar tissue, acts as a packing material between organs, providing support and flexibility. Adipose tissue, a type of loose connective tissue, stores fat and insulates the body. Dense connective tissue, with its tightly packed collagen fibers, forms strong structures like tendons and ligaments, which connect muscles to bones and bones to each other, respectively.

Cartilage is a flexible yet strong connective tissue found in joints, the ear, the nose, and the respiratory tract. It provides cushioning and support, allowing smooth movement at joints and maintaining the shape of structures like the ear and nose. Bone, a rigid connective tissue, forms the skeleton, providing structural support, protection for internal organs, and a site for muscle attachment. Blood, considered a connective tissue due to its origin in the bone marrow and its role in transport and immune function, circulates through the body, delivering oxygen and nutrients to cells and removing waste products.

Muscle tissue is specialized for contraction and movement. There are three types of muscle tissue: skeletal, cardiac, and smooth. Skeletal muscle tissue is attached to bones and is responsible for voluntary movements. It is composed of long, cylindrical cells with multiple nuclei and a striated appearance due to the organized arrangement of contractile proteins. These muscles are under conscious control, allowing precise and powerful movements.

Cardiac muscle tissue is found only in the heart. It is also striated but differs from skeletal muscle in that its cells are branched and interconnected, forming a network that allows coordinated contractions. Cardiac muscle cells have a single nucleus and are connected by intercalated discs, which facilitate the synchronized contraction of the heart, ensuring efficient blood pumping.

Smooth muscle tissue is found in the walls of internal organs, such as the stomach, intestines, blood vessels, and the bladder. Unlike skeletal and cardiac muscle, smooth muscle cells are spindle-shaped, lack striations, and have a single central nucleus. Smooth muscle contractions are involuntary and controlled by the autonomic nervous system, regulating processes like digestion, blood flow, and the expulsion of urine.

Nervous tissue is specialized for communication and control. It consists of neurons, which transmit electrical signals, and glial cells, which provide support and protection for neurons. Neurons are the functional units of the nervous system, capable of receiving, processing, and transmitting information. Each neuron has a cell body, dendrites, and an axon. Dendrites receive signals from other neurons, while the axon transmits signals to other neurons, muscles, or glands. This intricate network of neurons enables the nervous system to coordinate bodily functions, process sensory information, and enable thought and emotion.

Glial cells, or neuroglia, support neurons in various ways. They provide structural support, regulate the extracellular environment, facilitate signal transmission, and participate in the repair and maintenance of nervous tissue. Different types of glial cells perform specific functions; for instance, astrocytes maintain the blood-brain barrier, oligodendrocytes and Schwann cells produce myelin to insulate axons, and microglia act as immune cells within the nervous system.

The classification of tissues extends beyond their cellular composition to their roles in the body, reflecting the complexity and specialization required for the diverse functions of multicellular organisms. Each tissue type plays a crucial role in maintaining the body's homeostasis and overall health.

Understanding tissue classification is essential for many fields, including medicine, biology, and physiology. It aids in diagnosing diseases, developing treatments, and advancing research into how the body functions. For instance, recognizing the differences between benign and malignant tumors involves understanding the tissue origin and characteristics of the cells involved. Similarly, regenerative medicine and tissue engineering rely on knowledge of tissue structure and function to develop new therapies for repairing or replacing damaged tissues.

Epithelial Tissue: Structure and Function

Epithelial tissue is one of the four primary types of tissues in the human body, playing a vital role in covering surfaces, lining cavities, and forming glands. Its structure and function are intricately linked, allowing it to serve as a protective barrier, facilitate absorption and secretion, and provide sensory functions. Understanding epithelial tissue's unique characteristics and diverse functions provides insights into its critical role in maintaining the body's integrity and health.

Epithelial tissue is characterized by closely packed cells with minimal extracellular material, forming continuous sheets that cover surfaces and line cavities. This tight cellular arrangement is essential for its protective function, creating a barrier against physical, chemical, and microbial threats. Epithelial cells are anchored to a basement membrane, a specialized extracellular matrix that provides structural support and regulates cell behavior. The basement membrane separates the epithelium from underlying connective tissue, ensuring stability and facilitating nutrient exchange.

Epithelial cells exhibit polarity, meaning they have distinct apical and basal surfaces. The apical surface faces the external environment or a body cavity, while the basal surface attaches to the basement membrane. This polarity is crucial for the directional movement of substances across the epithelial layer. The apical surface often features specialized structures, such as microvilli or cilia, that enhance the tissue's functional capabilities. Microvilli increase surface area for absorption, as seen in the intestinal epithelium, while cilia help move mucus and trapped particles, as observed in the respiratory tract.

Epithelial tissues are classified based on the number of cell layers and the shape of the cells. Simple epithelium consists of a single layer of cells, making it ideal for functions requiring thin barriers, such as diffusion and filtration. In contrast, stratified epithelium has multiple cell layers, providing added protection against abrasion and wear. Additionally, epithelial cells can be squamous (flat), cuboidal (cube-shaped), or columnar (tall and cylindrical), each shape contributing to the tissue's specific function.

Simple squamous epithelium, composed of a single layer of flat cells, is found in locations where rapid diffusion or filtration is necessary. For instance, this tissue lines the alveoli in the lungs, facilitating gas exchange between air and blood. It also forms the endothelium of blood vessels, allowing efficient nutrient and waste exchange. The thinness of simple squamous epithelium reduces the distance over which substances must diffuse, enhancing efficiency.

Simple cuboidal epithelium, consisting of a single layer of cube-shaped cells, is commonly found in glandular tissues and kidney tubules. In glands, it functions in secretion, producing and releasing substances such as hormones, enzymes, and sweat. In the kidneys, simple cuboidal cells are involved in absorption and secretion, playing a critical role in urine formation and the regulation of blood composition. The cuboidal shape provides a balance between surface area for absorption and volume for housing cellular machinery involved in secretion.

Simple columnar epithelium, with tall, cylindrical cells, lines the digestive tract from the stomach to the rectum. This tissue is specialized for absorption and secretion, with cells often containing microvilli to increase surface area. Goblet cells, interspersed among the columnar cells, secrete mucus that lubricates the intestinal lining and protects it from digestive enzymes. The height of columnar cells allows for the accommodation of numerous organelles involved in the complex processes of digestion and nutrient absorption.

Stratified squamous epithelium, composed of multiple layers of flat cells, provides robust protection against mechanical stress and abrasion. This tissue forms the outer layer of the skin (epidermis) and lines the oral cavity, esophagus, and vagina. In the skin, the outermost cells are keratinized, meaning they contain the protein keratin, which enhances water resistance and durability. The non-keratinized version, found in moist environments like the mouth and esophagus, retains its nuclei and remains flexible, accommodating various mechanical stresses.

Pseudostratified columnar epithelium appears to have multiple layers due to the varying positions of cell nuclei, but it is actually a single layer with all cells attached to the basement membrane. This tissue lines the respiratory tract, where ciliated cells and goblet cells work together to trap and move particles out of the airways. The presence of cilia helps clear mucus and debris, protecting the respiratory system from infection and maintaining clear air passages.

Transitional epithelium, also known as urothelium, is a specialized type of stratified epithelium found in the urinary bladder, ureters, and part of the urethra. This tissue is uniquely adapted to stretch and recoil, allowing the bladder to expand as it fills with urine and contract when it empties. Transitional epithelial cells can change shape, appearing cuboidal when relaxed and squamous when stretched, providing a flexible yet protective lining for the urinary tract.

Epithelial tissue also forms glands, which are classified as either exocrine or endocrine based on their method of secretion. Exocrine glands, such as sweat, salivary, and digestive glands, release their products onto epithelial surfaces or into ducts. Endocrine glands, including the thyroid and adrenal glands, secrete hormones directly into the bloodstream, where they travel to target organs and regulate various physiological processes.

The regenerative capacity of epithelial tissue is remarkable, allowing it to quickly repair damage and maintain its functions. Stem cells located in the basal layer of stratified epithelia continuously divide, producing new cells that migrate to the surface and replace those lost to wear and tear. This rapid turnover is particularly evident in the skin and the lining of the digestive tract, where epithelial cells are constantly exposed to harsh environments.

Epithelial tissue's role in health and disease is profound. Its barrier function protects against pathogens, toxins, and physical injury, while its absorptive and secretory activities are essential for nutrient uptake and waste elimination. Dysfunctions in epithelial tissue can lead to various medical conditions, including infections, inflammatory diseases, and cancers. For example, breaches in the epithelial barrier can allow pathogens to invade underlying tissues, leading to infections. Chronic inflammation can disrupt epithelial function, as seen in conditions like inflammatory bowel disease. Additionally, epithelial cells are the origin of many cancers, known as carcinomas, due to their high turnover rate and exposure to environmental carcinogens.

Research into epithelial tissue has advanced our understanding of its biology and opened new avenues for medical treatments. Studies on epithelial cell behavior, regeneration, and responses to injury have led to innovations in wound healing, cancer therapy, and regenerative medicine. For instance, bioengineered skin grafts and cultured epithelial cells are used to treat burns and chronic wounds, offering new hope for patients with severe tissue damage.

Connective Tissue: Types and Roles

Connective tissue is a fundamental component of the human body, providing structural support, connecting different tissues, and playing roles in protection, insulation, and transportation. Unlike epithelial tissue, which is characterized by tightly packed cells, connective tissue is defined by its abundant extracellular matrix, which can vary greatly in composition and function. This diversity allows connective tissue to fulfill a wide range of roles essential for maintaining the body's integrity and function.

Connective tissue can be broadly classified into several types, each with distinct characteristics and functions. The primary types include loose connective tissue, dense connective tissue, cartilage, bone, blood, and lymph. Each type has specialized cells and an extracellular matrix tailored to its specific role.

Loose connective tissue, also known as areolar tissue, is the most widespread type of connective tissue in the body. It acts as a packing material, filling spaces between organs and providing a cushion to protect them. The extracellular matrix of loose connective tissue is composed of a gel-like ground substance with loosely arranged fibers, including collagen, elastic, and reticular fibers. The cells found in loose connective tissue include fibroblasts, which produce fibers and ground substance, as well as immune cells like macrophages and mast cells that defend against pathogens.

One of the most notable functions of loose connective tissue is its role in supporting epithelial tissues. It forms the lamina propria, a layer of connective tissue that underlies and nourishes the epithelium in mucous membranes. This connection is vital for maintaining the health and function of epithelial cells, as the loose connective tissue provides nutrients and removes waste products. Additionally, the flexibility and resilience of loose connective tissue allow it to absorb shock and accommodate movements in various parts of the body.

Dense connective tissue, in contrast, is characterized by a higher density of fibers, primarily collagen, which provides significant strength and resistance to stretching. There are two main types of dense connective tissue: dense regular and dense irregular. Dense regular connective tissue has parallel collagen fibers, making it well-suited for structures that require unidirectional tensile strength, such as tendons and ligaments. Tendons connect muscles to bones, transmitting the force generated by muscle contraction to produce movement, while ligaments connect bones to other bones, stabilizing joints and preventing excessive movement.

Dense irregular connective tissue, on the other hand, has collagen fibers arranged in various directions, providing multidirectional strength. This tissue type is found in areas subjected to stress from multiple directions, such as the dermis of the skin, the fibrous capsules surrounding organs, and the protective coverings of muscles and nerves. The collagen fibers in dense irregular connective tissue form a mesh-like network, distributing mechanical stress and preventing tissue damage.

Cartilage is a specialized type of connective tissue that provides flexible support and cushioning in joints. It has a firm, gel-like extracellular matrix rich in proteoglycans and collagen fibers, which give it both strength and elasticity. There are three types of cartilage: hyaline, elastic, and fibrocartilage. Hyaline cartilage, the most common type, covers the ends of long bones in joints, reducing friction and absorbing shock during movement. It also forms the embryonic skeleton, which is later replaced by bone, and is found in the respiratory tract, where it maintains the shape of structures like the trachea and bronchi.

Elastic cartilage contains a higher proportion of elastic fibers, making it more flexible than hyaline cartilage. This type is found in structures that require both strength and flexibility, such as the external ear and the epiglottis, which covers the larynx during swallowing to prevent food from entering the airway. Fibrocartilage, the toughest type, contains dense bundles of collagen fibers, providing great tensile strength and resistance to compression. It is found in intervertebral discs, which cushion the vertebrae in the spine, and in the menisci of the knee, which absorb shock and stabilize the joint.

Bone is a rigid, mineralized connective tissue that provides structural support, protects vital organs, and serves as a reservoir for minerals like calcium and phosphorus. The extracellular matrix of bone is composed of collagen fibers and hydroxyapatite crystals, which give bone its strength and hardness. Bone cells, or osteocytes, are embedded in this matrix and maintain bone tissue. There are two types of bone tissue: compact and spongy. Compact bone forms the dense outer layer of bones, providing strength for weight-bearing, while spongy bone, found in the interior, has a porous structure that reduces weight and contains bone marrow, where blood cells are produced.

Blood is a unique type of connective tissue with a liquid extracellular matrix called plasma. Plasma contains water, proteins, nutrients, hormones, and waste products. Suspended in the plasma are cellular components, including red blood cells, which transport oxygen; white blood cells, which fight infection; and platelets, which are involved in blood clotting. Blood serves as a transport system, delivering oxygen and nutrients to tissues, removing waste products, and distributing hormones throughout the body. It also plays a crucial role in immune defense and temperature regulation.

Lymph, another fluid connective tissue, circulates through the lymphatic system. It is derived from interstitial fluid, which surrounds tissue cells, and contains white blood cells, particularly lymphocytes, that are essential for immune responses. Lymphatic vessels collect lymph and return it to the bloodstream, maintaining fluid balance and filtering out pathogens and debris through lymph nodes.

Adipose tissue, or fat tissue, is a specialized form of loose connective tissue that stores energy, insulates the body, and cushions organs. Adipocytes, or fat cells, are the primary cell type in adipose tissue, and they store triglycerides, which can be broken down for energy during periods of fasting or increased energy demand. Adipose tissue is found beneath the skin, around internal organs, and in bone marrow. Beyond energy storage, adipose tissue secretes hormones and cytokines that regulate metabolism, inflammation, and other physiological processes.

The extracellular matrix of connective tissue is a dynamic environment that not only provides structural support but also influences cell behavior. Various proteins, such as collagen, elastin, and fibronectin, interact with cells through receptors on their surfaces, affecting cell adhesion, migration, proliferation, and differentiation. This interaction is crucial during development, wound healing, and tissue repair, where connective tissue cells and matrix components work together to restore tissue integrity.

Connective tissue disorders can arise from genetic mutations, autoimmune reactions, or environmental factors, leading to a wide range of diseases. For example, Marfan syndrome is a genetic disorder affecting the connective tissue protein fibrillin, resulting in weakened blood vessels, skeletal abnormalities, and eye problems. Rheumatoid arthritis is an autoimmune disease in which the immune system attacks the synovium, a specialized connective tissue in joints, causing inflammation, pain, and joint destruction. Scurvy, caused by vitamin C deficiency, impairs collagen synthesis, leading to weakened connective tissue, bleeding gums, and poor wound healing.

Advances in medical research and biotechnology have led to innovative treatments for connective tissue disorders. Tissue engineering techniques, such as the use of scaffolds and stem cells, aim to repair or replace damaged connective tissue. For instance, engineered cartilage and bone grafts are being developed to treat injuries and degenerative diseases. Additionally, understanding the molecular mechanisms underlying connective tissue function and pathology has paved the way for targeted therapies that modulate the immune response, promote tissue regeneration, and alleviate symptoms.

Muscle Tissue: Mechanisms of Contraction

Muscle tissue is a remarkable component of the human body, enabling movement, maintaining posture, and generating heat through the process of contraction. Understanding the mechanisms of muscle contraction provides insight into how the body performs everyday activities and responds to physical demands. There are three types of muscle tissue: skeletal, cardiac, and smooth, each with distinct structures and functions, but all relying on similar fundamental principles of contraction.

Skeletal muscle, the most abundant type, is responsible for voluntary movements and is attached to bones by tendons. It is composed of long, cylindrical cells called muscle fibers, which are multinucleated and striated. The striations, or stripes, are due to the regular arrangement of myofibrils within the fibers. Myofibrils are composed of repeating units called sarcomeres, the basic functional units of muscle contraction. Each sarcomere contains thick filaments of the protein myosin and thin filaments of the protein actin, arranged in a specific pattern that allows them to slide past one another during contraction.

The process of muscle contraction begins with a nerve impulse, or action potential, initiated in the motor cortex of the brain and transmitted through motor neurons to the muscle fibers. When the action potential reaches the neuromuscular junction, it triggers the release of the neurotransmitter acetylcholine (ACh) into the synaptic cleft. ACh binds to receptors on the muscle fiber's plasma membrane, or sarcolemma, causing ion channels to open and sodium ions to enter the cell. This depolarizes the sarcolemma and generates an action potential that travels along the membrane and down into the muscle fiber via structures called T-tubules.

The action potential in the T-tubules triggers the release of calcium ions from the sarcoplasmic reticulum, an internal storage site for calcium within the muscle fiber. Calcium ions bind to the protein troponin on the thin filaments, causing a conformational change that moves the protein tropomyosin away from binding sites on actin. This allows the myosin heads on the thick filaments to attach to the exposed binding sites on actin, forming cross-bridges.

The formation of cross-bridges is followed by the power stroke, a process in which the myosin heads pivot and pull the thin filaments toward the center of the sarcomere. This movement shortens the sarcomere, and consequently the entire muscle fiber, producing contraction. ATP, the energy currency of the cell, is required for the myosin heads to detach from actin and re-cock for another power stroke. As long as calcium ions remain elevated and ATP is available, the cycle of cross-bridge formation and power strokes continues, resulting in sustained muscle contraction.

Cardiac muscle, found exclusively in the heart, shares some structural similarities with skeletal muscle but also has unique features that allow it to function efficiently as a pump. Cardiac muscle fibers are striated like skeletal muscle fibers but are shorter, branched, and connected end-to-end by specialized junctions called intercalated discs. These discs contain gap junctions and desmosomes, which facilitate the rapid spread of electrical signals and mechanical force across the heart muscle, ensuring coordinated contractions.

The contraction of cardiac muscle is initiated by the heart's intrinsic pacemaker cells in the sinoatrial (SA) node, which generate rhythmic action potentials. These action potentials spread through the atria, causing them to contract, and then to the atrioventricular (AV) node, where there is a brief delay. From the AV node, the action potentials travel through the bundle of His, bundle branches, and Purkinje fibers, leading to the coordinated contraction of the ventricles. The mechanism of contraction at the cellular level in cardiac muscle is similar to that in skeletal muscle, involving the release of calcium ions and the interaction of actin and myosin filaments.

Smooth muscle is found in the walls of hollow organs such as the intestines, blood vessels, and the bladder. Unlike skeletal and cardiac muscle, smooth muscle is not striated because its actin and myosin filaments are arranged in a less orderly fashion. Smooth muscle cells are spindle-shaped and have a single nucleus. Contraction in smooth muscle is typically involuntary and can be triggered by a variety of stimuli, including neural input, hormones, and local chemical changes.

In smooth muscle, the mechanism of contraction involves the interaction of actin and myosin filaments, but the regulatory proteins and signaling pathways differ from those in striated muscle. Calcium ions play a central role in smooth muscle contraction, but instead of binding to troponin, they bind to a protein called calmodulin. The calcium-calmodulin complex activates myosin light-chain kinase, an enzyme that phosphorylates the myosin light chains, allowing myosin to bind to actin and initiate contraction. The process is slower and more sustained than in skeletal muscle, enabling smooth muscle to maintain tension for extended periods with less energy expenditure.

The contraction and relaxation of muscle tissues are finely regulated processes that ensure the body's movements are smooth and coordinated. Several factors influence muscle contraction, including the frequency of nerve impulses, the availability of calcium ions, and the energy status of the muscle fibers. For instance, during high-intensity exercise, the increased demand for ATP can lead to muscle fatigue if the energy supply cannot keep pace with consumption. Additionally, the removal of calcium ions from the sarcoplasm, either by reuptake into the sarcoplasmic reticulum or extrusion from the cell, is crucial for muscle relaxation.

Muscle tissue can adapt to various physical demands through processes such as hypertrophy and hyperplasia. Hypertrophy, the increase in muscle fiber size, occurs in response to resistance training and involves the synthesis of additional myofibrils and other cellular components. Hyperplasia, the increase in the number of muscle fibers, is less common in humans but can contribute to muscle growth under certain conditions. Regular exercise and proper nutrition are essential for maintaining muscle health and function, as they provide the stimuli and building blocks needed for muscle repair and growth.

Muscle tissue also has remarkable regenerative capabilities, particularly skeletal muscle, which can repair itself after injury. Satellite cells, a type of stem cell located between the sarcolemma and the basal lamina of muscle fibers, play a key role in muscle regeneration. Upon injury, satellite cells are activated, proliferate, and differentiate into new muscle fibers or fuse with existing fibers to aid in repair. However, severe or repeated injuries can overwhelm the regenerative capacity of muscle tissue, leading to fibrosis and impaired function.

Understanding the mechanisms of muscle contraction not only sheds light on how the body performs physical tasks but also has important implications for medical science and rehabilitation. Conditions such as muscular dystrophy, myasthenia gravis, and heart failure involve disruptions in normal muscle function and highlight the need for targeted therapies. Advances in molecular biology and biotechnology hold promise for developing new treatments that can enhance muscle repair, improve function, and alleviate the symptoms of muscle-related diseases.

Nervous Tissue: Signal Transmission

Nervous tissue is the cornerstone of the nervous system, responsible for transmitting signals throughout the body and enabling complex processes such as thought, sensation, and movement. This intricate system comprises neurons, the primary signaling cells, and glial cells, which provide support and protection. Understanding how nervous tissue transmits signals offers a glimpse into the remarkable functionality of the brain and peripheral nervous system.

Neurons, the fundamental units of nervous tissue, come in various shapes and sizes but share common features. Each neuron consists of a cell body (soma), dendrites, and an axon. The cell body contains the nucleus and metabolic machinery necessary for the cell's survival and function. Dendrites extend from the cell body and receive signals from other neurons or sensory cells. The axon, a long, slender projection, transmits signals to other neurons, muscles, or glands.

The transmission of signals within a neuron is an electrical process called an action potential. It begins when a neuron receives a sufficient stimulus, causing a rapid change in the electrical charge across its membrane. Neurons maintain a resting membrane potential, typically around -70 millivolts (mV), due to the distribution of ions, particularly sodium (Na+) and potassium (K+), across the membrane. This potential is maintained by the sodium-potassium pump, which actively transports Na+ out of and K+ into the cell.

When a neuron is stimulated, voltage-gated sodium channels open, allowing Na+ to rush into the cell. This influx of positive ions depolarizes the membrane, making the inside of the cell less negative. If the depolarization reaches a critical threshold, usually around -55 mV, an action potential is triggered. The action potential is an all-or-nothing event, meaning it either occurs fully or not at all.

During the action potential, the membrane potential rapidly rises to around +30 mV as more Na+ channels open. This depolarization phase is followed by the repolarization phase, where voltage-gated potassium channels open, allowing K+ to flow out of the cell. The efflux of K+ restores the membrane potential to a negative value. After repolarization, the membrane briefly becomes hyperpolarized, more negative than the resting potential, before returning to its resting state.

The action potential travels along the axon to the axon terminals, a process known as propagation. In myelinated neurons, the axon is covered by a fatty sheath called myelin, produced by glial cells (Schwann cells in the peripheral nervous system and oligodendrocytes in the central nervous system). Myelin insulates the axon and allows the action potential to jump between gaps in the sheath called nodes of Ranvier, a process known as saltatory conduction. This significantly increases the speed of signal transmission compared to unmyelinated axons.

When the action potential reaches the axon terminals, it triggers the release of chemical messengers called neurotransmitters. The transmission of signals between neurons occurs at specialized junctions called synapses. A synapse consists of the presynaptic terminal (axon terminal of the transmitting neuron), the synaptic cleft (a small gap between the neurons), and the postsynaptic membrane (dendrite or cell body of the receiving neuron).

The arrival of an action potential at the presynaptic terminal causes voltage-gated calcium channels to open, allowing Ca2+ to enter the terminal. The influx of calcium ions prompts synaptic vesicles containing neurotransmitters to fuse with the presynaptic membrane and release their contents into the synaptic cleft. The neurotransmitters diffuse across the cleft and bind to specific receptors on the postsynaptic membrane, leading to either excitation or inhibition of the postsynaptic neuron.

Excitatory neurotransmitters, such as glutamate, bind to receptors that open ion channels, allowing positive ions (e.g., Na+) to enter the postsynaptic neuron. This depolarizes the membrane and increases the likelihood of triggering an action potential. Inhibitory neurotransmitters, like gamma-aminobutyric acid (GABA), bind to receptors that open channels for negative ions (e.g., chloride, Cl-) or cause the efflux of positive ions (e.g., K+), hyperpolarizing the membrane and decreasing the likelihood of an action potential.

The precise effects of neurotransmitters depend on the types of receptors present on the postsynaptic membrane and the subsequent intracellular signaling pathways activated. Some neurotransmitters, such as acetylcholine, can have both excitatory and inhibitory effects depending on the receptor subtype they bind to. The balance between excitatory and inhibitory signals is crucial for proper nervous system function and regulation of activities like muscle contraction, hormone release, and mood.

The termination of neurotransmitter action is essential to prevent continuous stimulation or inhibition. This can occur through reuptake, where neurotransmitters are absorbed back into the presynaptic neuron, enzymatic degradation, where enzymes in the synaptic cleft break down neurotransmitters, or diffusion away from the synapse.

Glial cells, although not directly involved in signal transmission, play vital roles in maintaining the environment necessary for neurons to function effectively. Astrocytes, a type of glial cell, regulate the extracellular ion concentration, remove neurotransmitters from the synaptic cleft, and provide metabolic support to neurons. Microglia act as the immune cells of the central nervous system, protecting it from pathogens and clearing debris. The interplay between neurons and glial cells ensures the stability and efficiency of signal transmission.

Signal transmission in the nervous system underlies all aspects of human behavior, from simple reflexes to complex cognitive functions. Reflex arcs, for example, demonstrate the rapid and automatic nature of some neural responses. In a reflex arc, sensory neurons detect a stimulus and transmit the information to the spinal cord, where interneurons process it and immediately send signals to motor neurons, resulting in a quick, involuntary response.

Higher-order brain functions, such as learning and memory, involve more intricate neural circuits and synaptic plasticity. Synaptic plasticity refers to the ability of synapses to strengthen or weaken over time in response to activity levels. Long-term potentiation (LTP) and long-term depression (LTD) are key mechanisms of synaptic plasticity. LTP, often associated with learning and memory, involves the persistent strengthening of synapses based on recent patterns of activity, while LTD results in the weakening of synapses.

The nervous system's ability to adapt through synaptic plasticity highlights its dynamic nature. This adaptability is crucial for rehabilitation following neural injuries. For instance, after a stroke, which may damage parts of the brain, neural plasticity can aid in recovery by allowing other brain regions to compensate for lost functions. Rehabilitation therapies often focus on stimulating neural plasticity through repetitive, task-specific exercises.

Understanding the principles of signal transmission in nervous tissue also has significant implications for medical science. Disorders such as epilepsy, multiple sclerosis, and Parkinson's disease involve disruptions in normal neural signaling. Epilepsy is characterized by excessive and abnormal neural activity, leading to seizures. Multiple sclerosis involves the degeneration of myelin, impairing signal transmission. Parkinson's disease is associated with the loss of dopamine-producing neurons, leading to motor and cognitive deficits.

Advances in neuroscience and technology are paving the way for new treatments and interventions. Deep brain stimulation (DBS), for example, involves the implantation of electrodes in specific brain regions to modulate neural activity and alleviate symptoms of movement disorders. Neuroprosthetics, devices that interface with the nervous system, offer promise for restoring lost functions, such as enabling paralyzed individuals to control prosthetic limbs through neural signals.

Chapter 4

The Integumentary System

Structure and Function of the Skin

The skin, the body's largest organ, serves as a protective barrier while performing a multitude of essential functions. Comprising three primary layers—the epidermis, dermis, and hypodermis—each plays a unique role in maintaining the skin's integrity and overall health. Understanding the structure and function of the skin is crucial for recognizing its importance in safeguarding internal organs, regulating body temperature, and facilitating sensation.

The outermost layer, the epidermis, is a dynamic and multi-layered structure. It consists primarily of keratinocytes, cells that produce keratin, a tough and protective protein. The epidermis itself is divided into five strata: the stratum corneum, stratum lucidum, stratum granulosum, stratum spinosum, and stratum basale. Each layer has distinct characteristics and functions.

The stratum corneum, the outermost layer, is composed of dead keratinized cells that form a durable and waterproof barrier. These cells are continuously shed and replaced by new cells from the underlying layers. Just below, the stratum lucidum is found in thicker skin areas such as the palms and soles. It provides an additional layer of protection and is characterized by its clear appearance.

Moving deeper, the stratum granulosum contains keratinocytes that are beginning to die and accumulate keratohyalin granules, which contribute to the formation of the stratum corneum. The stratum spinosum, also known as the "spiny layer" due to the appearance of its cells under a microscope, plays a vital role in providing strength and flexibility to the skin. This layer is rich in desmosomes, structures that anchor cells together.

The deepest layer of the epidermis, the stratum basale, is where new keratinocytes are generated through mitosis. This layer also contains melanocytes, which produce melanin, the pigment responsible for skin color. Melanin provides protection against ultraviolet (UV) radiation by absorbing and dissipating harmful rays. The stratum basale is crucial for the continuous renewal of the epidermis, ensuring the skin remains resilient and capable of performing its protective functions.

Beneath the epidermis lies the dermis, a thicker and more complex layer composed of connective tissue. The dermis is divided into two regions: the papillary dermis and the reticular dermis. The papillary dermis, the uppermost part, consists of loose connective tissue with finger-like projections called dermal papillae. These projections interlock with the epidermis, strengthening the connection between the two layers and increasing the surface area for nutrient exchange.

The reticular dermis, found below the papillary dermis, is composed of dense irregular connective tissue, providing strength and elasticity to the skin. This layer contains collagen and elastin fibers, which help the skin withstand stretching and resist mechanical stress. Embedded within the dermis are various structures, including blood vessels, lymphatic vessels, nerves, and sensory receptors. These components play vital roles in thermoregulation, immune response, and sensation.

Hair follicles, sebaceous glands, and sweat glands are also located within the dermis. Hair follicles are responsible for producing hair, which provides additional protection and sensory input. Sebaceous glands secrete sebum, an oily substance that lubricates and waterproofs the skin and hair. Sweat glands, of which there are two types—eccrine and apocrine—are involved in thermoregulation and waste excretion. Eccrine glands are distributed throughout the body and produce a watery sweat, while apocrine glands, found in specific areas such as the armpits and groin, produce a thicker, milky sweat.

The deepest layer of the skin, the hypodermis (or subcutaneous layer), consists primarily of adipose tissue and loose connective tissue. This layer provides insulation, cushioning, and energy storage. The hypodermis anchors the skin to underlying structures such as muscles and bones, allowing for flexibility and movement. It also contains larger blood vessels and nerves that supply the skin and deeper tissues.

The skin's ability to regulate body temperature is a critical function, achieved through a combination of mechanisms. When the body overheats, blood vessels in the dermis dilate, increasing blood flow to the skin's surface and facilitating heat loss through radiation. Sweat production by eccrine glands increases, and as sweat evaporates from the skin's surface, it cools the body. Conversely, when the body is exposed to cold, blood vessels constrict, reducing blood flow to the skin and minimizing heat loss. The contraction of arrector pili muscles, attached to hair follicles, causes hair to stand upright, trapping an insulating layer of air close to the skin.

In addition to temperature regulation, the skin serves as a sensory organ, allowing us to perceive touch, pressure, pain, and temperature. Sensory receptors in the dermis, such as Meissner's corpuscles and Pacinian corpuscles, detect light touch and deep pressure, respectively. Free nerve endings in the skin respond to pain and temperature changes, providing vital information to the brain about the external environment.

The skin also plays an essential role in the immune system. Langerhans cells, found in the epidermis, are specialized dendritic cells that capture and present antigens to T-cells, initiating an immune response. The skin acts as a physical barrier to pathogens, preventing their entry into the body. Additionally, the acidic pH of the skin's surface and the presence of antimicrobial peptides create an inhospitable environment for many microorganisms.

Wound healing is another critical function of the skin. When the skin is injured, a complex and well-coordinated process begins to restore its integrity. The wound healing process can be divided into four phases: hemostasis, inflammation, proliferation, and remodeling. During hemostasis, blood vessels constrict, and a clot forms to stop bleeding. The inflammation phase involves the recruitment of immune cells to the wound site to clear debris and fight infection. In the proliferation phase, new tissue forms as fibroblasts produce collagen and other extracellular matrix components. Finally, during remodeling, the newly formed tissue matures and reorganizes, restoring the skin's strength and function.

The skin's structure and function can be influenced by various internal and external factors. Age, genetics, and hormones play significant roles in determining skin characteristics and susceptibility to conditions such as acne, eczema, and psoriasis. External factors, including UV radiation, pollution, and lifestyle choices, can impact skin health. Prolonged exposure to UV radiation, for example, can lead to photoaging, characterized by wrinkles, pigmentation changes, and an increased risk of skin cancer. Protective measures such as using sunscreen, wearing protective clothing, and avoiding excessive sun exposure are essential for maintaining skin health.

Nutrition also plays a vital role in skin health. A balanced diet rich in vitamins, minerals, and antioxidants supports the skin's structural integrity and function. For instance, vitamin C is crucial for collagen synthesis, while vitamin E provides antioxidant protection. Adequate hydration is essential for maintaining the skin's moisture balance and preventing dryness.

Maintaining healthy skin requires a combination of good skincare practices and a healthy lifestyle. Regular cleansing, moisturizing, and protection from environmental stressors are fundamental steps in a skincare routine. Gentle cleansing removes dirt, oil, and impurities without stripping the skin of its natural oils. Moisturizing helps maintain the skin's hydration barrier, preventing dryness and irritation. Using products with ingredients suited to one's skin type can enhance these effects.

Accessory Structures: Hair, Nails, and Glands

Hair, nails, and glands, though often overlooked, are integral components of the integumentary system. Each accessory structure serves unique functions that contribute to our overall health and well-being. Understanding these structures not only illuminates their biological significance but also highlights how they enhance our daily lives.

Hair, a defining characteristic of mammals, is more than just a feature of personal appearance. It grows from follicles located in the dermis, with each follicle undergoing a cycle of growth, rest, and shedding. This cycle comprises three phases: anagen (growth), catagen (transitional), and telogen (resting). During the anagen phase, cells in the hair bulb divide rapidly, pushing the hair shaft up and out. This phase can last several years, determining the maximum length of hair. In the catagen phase, lasting a few weeks, hair growth slows, and the follicle shrinks. Finally, in the telogen phase, the hair rests for a few months before falling out, making way for new growth.

The structure of hair includes the hair shaft, the visible part, and the hair root, hidden beneath the skin. The hair shaft consists of three layers: the medulla, cortex, and cuticle. The medulla, the innermost layer, is composed of loosely packed cells and air spaces. The cortex, which makes up the bulk of the hair, contains tightly packed keratin fibers that provide strength and color. The outermost layer, the cuticle, consists of overlapping cells that protect the inner layers from damage.

Hair serves various functions, from providing thermal insulation to facilitating sensory perception. On the scalp, hair protects against UV radiation and helps retain heat. Eyebrows and eyelashes shield the eyes from debris and sweat, while nasal hair filters particles from the air we breathe. Body hair, though less prominent, plays a role in detecting light touches and changes in the environment, contributing to our sensory experience.

Nails, another accessory structure, protect the tips of our fingers and toes while enhancing our ability to manipulate objects. They grow from the nail matrix, a region of rapidly dividing cells located under the base of the nail. As new cells are produced, older cells are pushed out, hardening and forming the visible nail plate. This process is continuous, with fingernails growing about 3 millimeters per month and toenails growing more slowly.

The nail plate, composed of hardened keratin, is divided into three parts: the free edge, the nail body, and the nail root. The free edge extends beyond the fingertip and is often trimmed. The nail body is the visible, pinkish part of the nail, while the nail root is hidden under the cuticle. The cuticle, a thin layer of skin, protects the nail matrix from infection and damage.

Nails provide several benefits, including improving fine motor skills and protecting the sensitive tips of our digits. They enhance our ability to perform tasks requiring precision, such as picking up small objects, typing, and scratching. Additionally, nails can serve as indicators of overall health; changes in color, texture, or growth patterns may signal underlying medical conditions.

Glands in the skin, specifically sebaceous and sweat glands, play crucial roles in maintaining homeostasis and protecting the body. Sebaceous glands, located in the dermis, secrete sebum, an oily substance that lubricates and waterproofs the skin and hair. Sebum helps prevent dehydration by reducing water loss from the skin's surface and has antimicrobial properties that protect against pathogens. These glands are most abundant on the face and scalp, where they contribute to the natural oils that keep skin and hair healthy.

Sweat glands, of which there are two types—eccrine and apocrine—are essential for thermoregulation and waste excretion. Eccrine glands, distributed across most of the body, produce a watery sweat that helps cool the body when it evaporates from the skin's surface. These glands are particularly concentrated on the palms, soles, and forehead. Apocrine glands, found in areas with dense hair follicles such as the armpits and groin, produce a thicker, milky sweat. This sweat, initially odorless, can develop a characteristic smell when broken down by bacteria on the skin's surface.

The regulation of sweat production is a finely tuned process involving the nervous system. When body temperature rises, the hypothalamus in the brain signals the sweat glands to produce sweat. This response not only cools the body but also helps excrete waste products such as urea and salts. In stressful situations, the sympathetic nervous system activates eccrine glands, leading to sweaty palms and other areas, a response linked to the body's fight-or-flight mechanism.

Beyond their primary functions, these accessory structures also play roles in social and cultural contexts. Hair, for instance, is a significant aspect of personal identity and cultural expression. Hairstyles can signify belonging to a particular group, convey social status, or reflect individual personality. Throughout history, hair has been styled, colored, and adorned in myriad ways, highlighting its importance beyond mere biology.

Similarly, nails have cultural and aesthetic significance. Well-groomed nails are often associated with hygiene and attention to personal appearance. In many cultures, nail art and decoration have become forms of self-expression, with trends and styles evolving over time. The practice of manicuring and decorating nails dates back thousands of years, underscoring their enduring appeal.

Glands, though less visible, also have social implications. The production of body odor, regulated by apocrine glands, can affect social interactions and perceptions. Cultural attitudes towards body odor vary widely, with different societies adopting various practices to manage or mask it. Personal hygiene products, such as deodorants and antiperspirants, have become ubiquitous in many cultures, reflecting the desire to control body odor and maintain social norms.

Caring for these accessory structures involves a combination of good hygiene practices, proper nutrition, and attentive grooming. For hair, regular washing with suitable products, minimizing heat and chemical damage, and maintaining a balanced diet rich in vitamins and minerals can promote healthy growth and appearance. For nails, keeping them clean, trimmed, and moisturized helps prevent infections and breakage. Avoiding habits such as biting nails and using harsh chemicals can also protect nail health.

Maintaining healthy skin glands involves regular cleansing to remove excess oil and sweat, which can clog pores and lead to conditions such as acne. Using gentle skincare products and avoiding excessive scrubbing can help maintain the skin's natural balance. Staying hydrated and consuming a diet rich in nutrients supports the overall function of sebaceous and sweat glands.

Incorporating these practices into daily routines can enhance the health and appearance of hair, nails, and skin. Awareness of the functions and needs of these accessory structures empowers individuals to make informed choices about their care. By fostering a holistic approach to personal grooming and hygiene, we can better appreciate the intricate interplay between these structures and our overall well-being.

Skin Disorders and Diseases

Skin disorders and diseases, affecting millions worldwide, range from minor irritations to severe conditions impacting quality of life. Understanding these conditions is crucial to managing and preventing them. This chapter delves into common skin disorders and diseases, their causes, symptoms, and treatment options, providing practical advice for beginners navigating these often complex issues.

Acne, one of the most prevalent skin conditions, affects up to 85% of people at some point in their lives. It typically emerges during adolescence but can persist into adulthood. Acne develops when hair follicles become clogged with oil and dead skin cells, leading to whiteheads, blackheads, and pimples. Hormonal changes, particularly during puberty, trigger increased oil production, exacerbating acne. Other factors include genetics, diet, and stress.

Managing acne involves a combination of proper skincare, lifestyle adjustments, and medical treatments. Daily cleansing with a gentle, non-comedogenic cleanser helps remove excess oil and dirt. Over-the-counter treatments containing benzoyl peroxide or salicylic acid can reduce inflammation and clear pores. For persistent or severe acne, dermatologists may prescribe topical retinoids, antibiotics, or oral medications like isotretinoin. Maintaining a healthy diet, managing stress, and avoiding harsh skincare products can also mitigate acne symptoms.

Eczema, or atopic dermatitis, is another common skin disorder, characterized by red, itchy, and inflamed skin. It often appears in childhood but can affect individuals of any age. Eczema's exact cause remains unknown, but it is believed to result from a combination of genetic and environmental factors. Triggers such as allergens, irritants, stress, and weather changes can exacerbate symptoms.

Effective eczema management focuses on reducing symptoms and preventing flare-ups. Moisturizing regularly with emollients helps maintain the skin barrier and prevent dryness. Identifying and avoiding triggers, such as certain soaps, detergents, and fabrics, can minimize irritation. During flare-ups, topical corticosteroids and calcineurin inhibitors reduce inflammation and itching. Severe cases may require systemic treatments like oral corticosteroids or biologics. Additionally, maintaining a consistent skincare routine and practicing good hygiene can reduce eczema's impact on daily life.

Psoriasis, an autoimmune disease, causes rapid skin cell turnover, leading to thick, scaly patches of skin. These patches, or plaques, are often red and covered with silvery scales, and they can occur anywhere on the body. Psoriasis is a chronic condition with periods of remission and flare-ups, triggered by factors such as stress, infections, and certain medications. Genetics play a significant role in predisposition to psoriasis.

Treatment for psoriasis aims to slow cell turnover and reduce inflammation. Topical treatments, including corticosteroids, vitamin D analogs, and retinoids, can help manage mild to moderate cases. For more severe psoriasis, phototherapy or systemic medications like methotrexate, cyclosporine, and biologics may be prescribed. Lifestyle modifications, such as maintaining a healthy weight, reducing alcohol consumption, and avoiding smoking, can also improve symptoms and overall health.

Rosacea, a chronic skin condition, primarily affects the face, causing redness, swelling, and visible blood vessels. Flare-ups can trigger pimples and thickened skin, particularly on the nose. The exact cause of rosacea is unknown, but it is thought to involve a combination of genetic and environmental factors. Triggers include hot or cold weather, spicy foods, alcohol, and stress.

Managing rosacea involves identifying and avoiding triggers, using gentle skincare products, and protecting the skin from sun exposure. Topical treatments like metronidazole and azelaic acid, along with oral antibiotics such as doxycycline, can reduce inflammation and pimple formation. In some cases, laser therapy may be used to diminish visible blood vessels and redness. Consistent care and avoidance of known triggers are key to managing rosacea effectively.

Skin cancer, the most common form of cancer, arises from uncontrolled growth of abnormal skin cells. The primary types include basal cell carcinoma, squamous cell carcinoma, and melanoma. Basal cell carcinoma is the most common and least aggressive, while melanoma is less common but more dangerous due to its potential to spread to other parts of the body. Risk factors for skin cancer include excessive sun exposure, tanning bed use, fair skin, and a history of sunburns.

Prevention and early detection are vital in combating skin cancer. Regular use of broad-spectrum sunscreen with an SPF of 30 or higher, wearing protective clothing, and seeking shade can reduce the risk of UV damage. Monthly self-examinations and annual skin checks by a dermatologist help detect early signs of skin cancer. Treatment options vary depending on the type and stage of cancer, ranging from surgical removal and cryotherapy to radiation and targeted therapies for advanced cases.

Contact dermatitis, an inflammatory reaction to substances that come into contact with the skin, manifests as red, itchy, and sometimes blistered skin. It can be classified into two types: irritant contact dermatitis and allergic contact dermatitis. Irritant contact dermatitis occurs when the skin is damaged by irritants such as chemicals, detergents, or prolonged exposure to water. Allergic contact dermatitis results from an immune response to allergens like nickel, fragrances, or poison ivy.

Managing contact dermatitis involves identifying and avoiding the offending substance, using protective measures such as gloves, and applying topical corticosteroids to reduce inflammation and itching. In severe cases, oral corticosteroids or other immune-modulating medications may be necessary. Maintaining a healthy skin barrier with regular moisturization can also help prevent contact dermatitis.

Warts, caused by the human papillomavirus (HPV), are benign growths that can appear anywhere on the skin. Common types include common warts, plantar warts, and flat warts. Warts are spread through direct contact with the virus, often occurring in areas of broken skin. Though generally harmless, warts can be unsightly and sometimes painful, particularly when located on weight-bearing areas like the soles of the feet.

Treatment options for warts include over-the-counter solutions containing salicylic acid, which gradually dissolve the wart tissue. Cryotherapy, or freezing the wart with liquid nitrogen, is another common method. For persistent or resistant warts, dermatologists may use laser treatment, immunotherapy, or minor surgical procedures. Maintaining good hygiene and avoiding direct contact with warts can help prevent their spread.

Fungal infections, such as athlete's foot, ringworm, and yeast infections, thrive in warm, moist environments. These infections often affect areas like the feet, groin, and under the breasts. Symptoms vary but typically include itching, redness, and scaling. Fungal infections can spread through direct contact with infected individuals or contaminated surfaces.

Effective management of fungal infections involves keeping affected areas clean and dry, using antifungal creams or powders, and avoiding sharing personal items like towels and footwear. In more severe cases, oral antifungal medications may be prescribed. Preventive measures include wearing breathable clothing, changing out of damp clothes promptly, and using moisture-wicking socks and shoes.

The Role of the Skin in Thermoregulation

The skin, our body's largest organ, plays a crucial role in thermoregulation, the process of maintaining a stable internal temperature despite external fluctuations. This remarkable ability is essential for our survival, allowing us to adapt to various environmental conditions and maintain homeostasis. Through a combination of physiological mechanisms and behavioral adaptations, the skin helps balance heat production and heat loss, ensuring our core temperature remains within a narrow, optimal range.

One of the primary ways the skin contributes to thermoregulation is through the regulation of blood flow. The skin contains a vast network of blood vessels that can dilate or constrict in response to temperature changes. When exposed to heat, the blood vessels in the skin dilate, a process known as vasodilation. This increases blood flow to the skin's surface, allowing heat to dissipate into the environment. Conversely, in cold conditions, the blood vessels constrict, or undergo vasoconstriction, reducing blood flow to the skin's surface and minimizing heat loss. This dynamic adjustment of blood flow is a key mechanism in temperature regulation.

Sweating is another critical function of the skin in thermoregulation. Sweat glands, particularly the eccrine glands, produce sweat in response to rising body temperatures. As sweat evaporates from the skin's surface, it absorbs heat, effectively cooling the body. This evaporative cooling is highly efficient and can significantly lower body temperature during intense physical activity or in hot environments. However, the effectiveness of sweating depends on factors such as humidity and air movement, which influence the rate of evaporation.

The skin also houses a complex network of nerve endings that detect changes in temperature. These thermoreceptors send signals to the hypothalamus, the brain region responsible for regulating body temperature. The hypothalamus then initiates appropriate responses to maintain thermal balance. For instance, if the body becomes too hot, the hypothalamus triggers sweating and vasodilation. If the body is too cold, it induces vasoconstriction and shivering, another mechanism for generating heat through muscle activity.

Behavioral adaptations complement these physiological mechanisms. When we feel hot, we instinctively seek shade, remove excess clothing, or drink cold fluids. Conversely, in cold environments, we layer clothing, seek shelter, or consume warm beverages. These behaviors, driven by our perception of temperature changes, enhance the skin's ability to regulate body temperature effectively.

The skin's role in thermoregulation is particularly evident during exercise. Physical activity generates significant heat due to increased metabolic activity in muscles. To prevent overheating, the body relies heavily on the skin's cooling mechanisms. Sweating becomes more pronounced, and blood flow to the skin increases to facilitate heat dissipation. This is why it's vital to stay hydrated during exercise, as dehydration can impair sweating and, consequently, thermoregulation, leading to heat-related illnesses such as heat exhaustion or heat stroke.

In addition to managing heat, the skin also plays a role in conserving warmth in cold conditions. The subcutaneous fat layer beneath the skin acts as an insulator, reducing heat loss. In response to cold, the skin's hair follicles contract, causing hairs to stand up, a response known as piloerection or "goosebumps." Although this reaction is more pronounced in animals with thick fur, it still provides some insulation in humans by trapping a thin layer of air close to the skin.

Certain populations, such as infants and the elderly, are more vulnerable to temperature extremes due to differences in skin structure and function. Infants have a higher surface area-to-body mass ratio and thinner skin, making them more susceptible to heat loss. Additionally, their sweat glands are not fully developed, reducing their ability to cool down through sweating. The elderly, on the other hand, often experience a decline in sweat gland function and blood vessel responsiveness, impairing their thermoregulatory capacity. Understanding these vulnerabilities underscores the importance of special care and monitoring for these groups during extreme temperatures.

Environmental factors can also impact the skin's thermoregulatory functions. High humidity levels, for instance, hinder the evaporation of sweat, reducing the effectiveness of cooling. Windy conditions, on the other hand, enhance heat loss by increasing the rate of sweat evaporation and convective heat transfer. Clothing choices can either support or hinder thermoregulation. Lightweight, breathable fabrics facilitate heat dissipation, while insulating layers trap heat and reduce heat loss, aiding in temperature maintenance in cold environments.

Certain medical conditions can disrupt the skin's ability to regulate temperature. For example, hyperhidrosis, characterized by excessive sweating, can lead to dehydration and impair cooling. Conversely, conditions like anhidrosis, where sweat production is insufficient, can result in overheating. Peripheral vascular diseases, which affect blood flow to the extremities, can also compromise thermoregulation, particularly in cold environments, increasing the risk of frostbite or hypothermia.

Advancements in wearable technology are providing new insights into the skin's role in thermoregulation. Devices that monitor skin temperature, sweat rate, and other physiological parameters can help individuals optimize their thermal comfort and performance. For athletes, such technology can inform hydration strategies and training regimens, while for outdoor workers, it can enhance safety by preventing heat-related illnesses.

Cultural practices and historical adaptations also highlight the skin's role in thermoregulation. Traditional clothing and architectural designs in different cultures reflect adaptations to local climates. For instance, loose, flowing garments in desert regions promote airflow and cooling, while tightly woven fabrics in colder climates provide insulation. These cultural adaptations, developed over generations, emphasize the importance of understanding and optimizing the skin's thermoregulatory functions.

As climate change leads to more frequent and severe temperature extremes, understanding the skin's role in thermoregulation becomes increasingly important. Rising temperatures and heatwaves pose significant health risks, particularly for vulnerable populations. Strategies to mitigate these risks include promoting public awareness about the importance of hydration, appropriate clothing, and recognizing the signs of heat-related illnesses. Community planning and infrastructure development can also enhance resilience, such as creating shaded areas and cooling centers in urban environments.

Wound Healing and Tissue Repair

Wound healing and tissue repair are fundamental processes that the body employs to restore integrity and function to damaged tissues. These complex and dynamic processes involve a series of overlapping stages, each characterized by specific cellular and molecular events. Understanding these stages provides valuable insights into how the body manages injuries and what can be done to support and enhance healing.

The initial response to tissue injury is the hemostasis phase, which begins immediately after the wound occurs. The primary goal during this phase is to stop bleeding and form a stable clot. Blood vessels constrict to reduce blood flow, and platelets aggregate at the injury site to form a temporary plug. These platelets release signaling molecules that attract additional platelets and initiate the coagulation cascade, resulting in the formation of a fibrin clot. This clot not only prevents further blood loss but also serves as a scaffold for incoming cells that will participate in the healing process.

Following hemostasis, the inflammatory phase sets in. This phase is characterized by the recruitment of immune cells to the wound site to clear debris, pathogens, and dead tissue. Neutrophils are among the first responders, arriving within hours to engulf and digest bacteria and damaged cells. They are soon followed by macrophages, which play a dual role: they continue the cleanup process through phagocytosis and secrete cytokines that orchestrate the next stages of healing. The inflammatory phase is essential for preventing infection and preparing the wound bed for tissue repair, but it must be carefully regulated to avoid excessive inflammation, which can impede healing.

The proliferation phase marks the period of active tissue formation and repair. This phase involves several key processes: angiogenesis, collagen deposition, granulation tissue formation, and epithelialization. Angiogenesis, the formation of new blood vessels, is crucial for supplying oxygen and nutrients to the healing tissue. Endothelial cells from existing blood vessels migrate to the wound site and form new capillary loops, creating a rich vascular network.

Fibroblasts, which are attracted to the wound by growth factors released during the inflammatory phase, begin to synthesize and deposit collagen. This protein provides structural support and strength to the new tissue. The collagen matrix forms the basis of granulation tissue, which fills the wound and serves as a foundation for further tissue development. At the same time, keratinocytes, the primary cells of the epidermis, migrate across the wound bed from the edges to re-establish the protective skin barrier in a process known as epithelialization.

The final phase of wound healing is remodeling, which can last for months or even years. During this phase, the newly formed tissue undergoes maturation and reorganization to restore normal function and appearance. Collagen fibers are realigned along tension lines to increase tensile strength, and the extracellular matrix is remodeled to remove excess components. Myofibroblasts, specialized cells that combine properties of fibroblasts and smooth muscle cells, play a key role in wound contraction, reducing the size of the wound as it heals. Although the remodeled tissue may never fully regain the strength and elasticity of uninjured skin, the result is a closed wound with restored barrier function.

Several factors can influence the efficiency and success of wound healing. These include the patient's overall health, age, nutrition, and the presence of underlying medical conditions. For instance, diabetes can impair wound healing by affecting blood flow and immune function, leading to chronic, non-healing wounds. Similarly, poor nutrition, particularly a lack of essential vitamins and proteins, can delay the healing process by depriving the body of the building blocks needed for tissue repair.

Chronic wounds represent a significant challenge in wound care. These wounds, which fail to progress through the normal stages of healing, often remain stuck in the inflammatory phase. Common examples include diabetic foot ulcers, pressure ulcers, and venous leg ulcers. Managing chronic wounds requires a multifaceted approach that addresses underlying issues, such as improving blood circulation, controlling infection, and optimizing wound care practices. Advanced therapies, such as growth factors, skin substitutes, and hyperbaric oxygen therapy, may also be employed to promote healing in these difficult cases.

Innovations in wound care continue to evolve, driven by a deeper understanding of the cellular and molecular mechanisms underlying tissue repair. One promising area of research is the use of stem cells to enhance healing. Stem cells have the potential to differentiate into various cell types needed for tissue repair and can secrete bioactive molecules that modulate the healing environment. Clinical trials are exploring the use of stem cell-based therapies for treating complex wounds and enhancing regeneration.

Another exciting development is the use of biomaterials and tissue engineering to create scaffolds that support and guide tissue regeneration. These scaffolds can be designed to mimic the natural extracellular matrix, providing a conducive environment for cell attachment, proliferation, and differentiation. By incorporating growth factors and other bioactive agents, these biomaterials can further enhance the healing process.

The role of dressings in wound care cannot be overlooked. Modern wound dressings are designed to create an optimal healing environment by maintaining moisture balance, protecting the wound from infection, and promoting tissue regeneration. Hydrocolloid, foam, and alginate dressings are among the many options available, each tailored to different types and stages of wounds. The choice of dressing depends on factors such as the wound's size, depth, exudate level, and presence of infection.

Patient education and involvement are also critical components of effective wound management. Patients need to understand the importance of adhering to treatment plans, maintaining good hygiene, and recognizing early signs of complications. Healthcare providers play a key role in educating patients and caregivers, offering guidance on wound care practices, and providing support throughout the healing process.

Lifestyle modifications can further support wound healing. Quitting smoking, for instance, can significantly improve healing outcomes, as smoking constricts blood vessels and reduces oxygen delivery to tissues. Regular exercise enhances circulation and overall health, while a balanced diet ensures the body has the necessary nutrients for repair. Stress management is also important, as chronic stress can negatively impact immune function and delay healing.

www.ingramcontent.com/pod-product-compliance
Lightning Source LLC
Chambersburg PA
CBHW071219130726

47998CB00002B/777